CHANGING THE NORM

"A Black Woman's Guide to Eating, Feeling and Looking Her Best"

Disclaimer

Every effort has been made to make all publications and products sold through this site or through phone and mail as complete and accurate as possible. However, there may be mistakes both typographical and in content. Therefore, this text should be used only as a general guide and not as the ultimate reference source.

The information presented in this publication is not intended as specific medical advice and is not a substitute for professional medical treatment or diagnosis.

The contents of this publication, including articles, graphics, images, and all other material, are for your private use and informational purposes only. If you have a medical emergency, do not rely on the content to treat your condition; call your doctor or go to a hospital immediately. The content is not intended to be professional medical advice, diagnosis, or treatment.

Always seek the advice of your physician or other qualified health professional for questions you have regarding any medical concerns or conditions.

Reliance on the content or any other information provided by Laticia "Action" Jackson or any of her employees, agents, authors or others providing content to this book is solely at your own risk. The content is provided on an "as is" basis.

Changing the "NORM"

"A Black Woman's Guide to Eating, Feeling and Looking Her Best"

Published in arrangement with
www.laticiaactionjackson.com

By

Laticia "Action" Jackson

2008 Fitness Olympian

Masters of Public Health (M.P.H.)

B.S. Exercise Science/Master Level Personal Trainer

Certified Lifestyle and Weight Management Specialist

Certified Corporate Wellness Coach

3-Time N.P.C. State Fitness Champion

© *2017 All rights reserved.*

Fitness Images by Jiame Rivera

Jar Studio.com

This book, or any parts thereof,

may not be reproduced in any

form without permission.

Visit our website at
www.laticiaactionjackson.com

Testimonies

"Laticia "Action" Jackson is a student of the game and a master of her craft."
Daryl Haley ~ Retired N.F.L New England Patriots

"Laticia Jackson is a fitness inspiration who walks the walk. Follow her lead and you're sure to change your body for the better."
Brad Schoenfeld, MS, CSCS ~ Author: Women's Home Workout Bible

---

"Undeniably the best fitness trainer I have ever had the privilege to interview or work with. She pushes you to be your best. Not only physically- and believe me she's tough. But internally which gives you the permission to be your best-mind, body and spirit!"
Mark Mathis ~ CW31 Good Day Sacramento

"One Dynamic Lady whose passion to succeed and make a difference has made her dynamic in all areas of her life."
Mike Lackner ~ Body Fitness-UK

"Every workout was earnest, extremely enjoyable and tailored to my personal needs allowing me to reach my maximum physical fitness level. Laticia was inspirational, motivating and I highly endorse her as a physical fitness trainer for anyone and everyone."
Lloyd C. ~ Colonel U.S.A.F., Dayton Ohio

"Working with Laticia Jackson as my personal trainer has been an empowering experience. She trains your body to achieve maximum performance, teaches your mind new fitness concepts and encourages your inner self to embrace and love the healthy person you are destined to be."
Sandra H. ~ California Police Dept., Sacramento, CA

TABLE OF CONTENTS

Dedication 1

Acknowledgments 3

Introduction 4

My Journey 6

Part 1: CHANGING THE NORM! 8

Chapter 1: Obesity, The Great Epidemic 9

Chapter 2: Is Your Confidence Killing You? 14

Chapter 3: Why Can't You Change? 18

Chapter 4: What's Your Motivation? 22

Chapter 5: Remove the Mask 25

Chapter 6: A Heart Beat Away 33

Chapter 7: Change Your Mind, Change Your Body 39

Chapter 8: 10 Days of Inner Discovery 44

Part 2: FUEL YOUR SUCCESS 55

Chapter 9: You Are What You Eat! 56

Chapter 10: Don't Believe the Hype 60

Chapter 11: Friend vs. Foe 64

Chapter 12: No More Dieting 66

Chapter 13: Protein the Building Blocks 68

Chapter 14: Fat Attack 74

Chapter 15: Carbs: The Energy Makers 81

Chapter 16: Tools for Success 97

Chapter 17: It's a Family Affair 101

Chapter 18: Feed the Machine 104

Part 3: YOUR FITNESS JOURNEY 125

Chapter 19: Let's Address the Barriers! 126

Chapter 20: I Can't Afford to Get Fit! 130

Chapter 21: 5 Steps to Get **CURVE**licious...132

Chapter 22: Before You Begin...152

Chapter 23: Learn The Principles and Terminology......................................165

Chapter 24: Social Hour is Over 168

Chapter 25: Gym Etiquette 101 171

Chapter 26: Cardio Fit...174

Chapter 27: Stretching Essentials 180

Chapter 28: Define Your Curves 185

About the Author... 242

Index.. 244

Dedication

Who is This Book Dedicated To?

This book is dedicated to the African American woman who desires the tools to EAT, FEEL, and LOOK her best.

This book is also dedicated to the African American woman, who says she's ready to change the statistic that acknowledges four out of five African American women are obese.

Why Did I Write This Book?

I believe there's a hunger and desire within many African American women to live a healthier lifestyle. However, there are few African American female role models represented in mainstream media or within the African American community that reflect the image of fitness and healthy living.

This is not an excuse or blame, rather, an awareness that it is essential for one to repeatedly see an example of healthy living in order to strive for it.

I Know Your Challenges

As an African American woman, I understand the challenges and cultural barriers that prevent many African American women from reaching a better state of health.

Therefore, it has become my mission to provide African American women with the tools to transform their health by providing evidence-based information in the areas of exercise, healthy nutrition and behavior change.

Why So Much Passion?

In my 20's I knew I wanted to change lives by empowering individuals with the tools to take control of their health. Therefore over the last 15 years I have acquired the knowledge, skills and abilities to provide you with researched and evidence-based information that when applied can assist you in reaching a state of optimal (satisfactory) health.

In the following chapters, I provide you with the tools to address risk factors such as poor nutrition, limited physical activity and stress that contribute to many chronic health problems such as obesity, type 2 diabetes, heart disease, hypertension and some forms of cancer that plague millions of African American women.

Throughout the following pages, I also encourage you to identify cultural and social barriers that contribute to how you see your body and healthy living.

It's my belief that through honest and transparent conversations, African American women CAN change the "NORM" and begin to see our bodies and healthy living from a new perspective.

Lifestyle behavior changes don't occur overnight, however, if you begin to make yourself and your health a priority you can create a healthier future one healthy decision at a time.

Will you JOIN me?

If your answer is yes, let's begin changing the "NORM"!

Love,

Laticia "Action "Jackson

2008 Fitness Olympian/Health & Fitness Expert/ MPH/ B.S. Exercise Science

Stay Fit,

Stay True,

Stay You!

Laticia "Action" Jackson

Acknowledgments

First and most importantly, I would like to thank my Creator for entrusting me with this vision. I am forever grateful for the gifts you have given me. May I always live a life that is pleasing and honorable in your sight. I love you and will always need you. You are amazing!

Mom, there are not enough words in the dictionary to describe how much I love you. Regardless of what life has brought my way, you have always been there to love me through my trials. A day without you is comparable to a day without the sun. You are my light and my best friend. I pray one day I will be a great mother just like you.

Dad, you have always been a silent strength in my life. I have inherited your tremendous work ethic and it has paid off in so many ways. You are a man of great character and integrity and I pray to one day marry a man with your morals and values. I look forward to our relationship growing. It's great to find out who I get my long arms from!

Yolanda, I would like to thank you for always being there for me. You are always just a call away. You are officially my human resource person. Your strength as a soldier, mother, sister, wife and friend is encouraging. May God give you all the desires of your heart and much more. I pray you learn to laugh more often; you know I do enough laughing for the both of us. You are a great big sister and I love you.

Shanta, we have been friends for as long as I can remember. Even though you have left me outside in the cold to get a donut, I will always love you. You are the true image of a wife and mother. You are selfless and I admire that about you. Your constant prayers, love, and encouragement, is priceless. You have a special place in my heart. I love you butterfly. Thanks for letting me be your little sister.

To my nieces and nephews, you bring so much joy to my life. It has been such a pleasure to be your auntie. Seeing each of you grow up brings joy to my heart. I love each of you.

To my brother-in-law's, thanks for loving my sisters and being great men.

Introduction

In a culture where being *"thick"* is often praised by both men and women, celebrated by R&B and Rap industries, it's hard not to embrace the curves and full figured frame of the African American woman. African American women are CURVY, SHAPELY and make no apologies for it!

What's the Problem?

It's possible you're wondering why African American women shouldn't feel great about their full framed bodies. Is there something wrong with African American women loving and embracing their voluptuous frames?

In most cases the answer is no, however, for the purpose of this book, the answer is yes and I will explain why! In the following chapters, I will explain why the voluptuous and curvy frame of many African American women can be dangerous and potentially deadly.

I will also explain how your environment can be hazardous to your health and more importantly, I will provide you with the tools to change the alarming statistic from the Centers for Disease Control (CDC) that acknowledges four out of five African American women are obese.

It is my hope that by exposing you to these truths, you will begin to understand the importance of achieving and maintaining a healthy body weight and take to heart the necessity of creating healthy lifestyle behaviors that can lead to better overall health for yourself, your community and your family.

Why Changing the "NORM"?

There are numerous health, wellness, fitness and nutrition books on the buyers' market, however, few of these books capture first-hand the struggles of being an African American woman who desires to get fit and healthy in a culture that doesn't promote healthy living on a regular basis.

As an African American woman, I understand the unique struggles, challenges and barriers that black women face and that's why I have chosen to write *"Changing the Norm - A Black Woman's Guide to Eating, Feeling and Looking HER Best."*

CHANGING THE NORM

Throughout the chapters of this book, you will discover the tools to create a new mindset about how you see yourself, your body and your health. I need to warn you: you won't find any information on how to diet in this book. Diets don't work. They are short-lived, unrealistic and expensive. Instead of learning how to diet, you will discover basic nutrition principles that teach you how to shop, prepare and cook healthy meals for yourself, your community and your family.

I won't recommend diet pills for weight loss. However, I will teach you how to identify your body type, how to properly exercise for your body type, and how to make yourself a priority in order to achieve a healthy body weight.

Healthy eating can seem boring when you have been raised in a culture where palate pleasing foods have been used to bring family and friends together for centuries. Therefore if you feel hesitant about healthy eating, I understand the fear of changing your food choices. I understand your concerns, however, allow me to place your fears about healthy eating to rest. Becoming healthy isn't about eating bland foods, it's about eating nutritious foods you enjoy and using healthy seasonings and fresh ingredients to add flavoring. I understand the importance of food in our culture, therefore within the following chapters I provide you with easy to prepare recipes for breakfast, lunch and dinner that will satisfy your taste buds, along with snacks that can be prepared in less than 5 minutes. I don't want you to get rid of the traditional foods you love; instead, I will show you how to cook traditional African American staples the healthy way!

Making the decision to change unhealthy lifestyle behaviors can seem overwhelming at first, but rest assured, you're not alone. I am here to walk with you step-by-step in your health and fitness journey. Don't take this journey alone, grab a few of your girlfriends and take them with you on this journey. It's my belief, sisters who get healthier together, live a longer life together!

Are ready to CHANGE the "NORM"? If you are, let the changing begin!

My Journey

When Did My Passion Begin?

I'm often asked why I am so passionate about helping others become healthy. My response? It was a part of my creator's plan. I just realized it at the age of 19.

How Did My Love for Health and Fitness Begin?

In 2001, at the age of 19, I entered the United States Air Force with the hopes of making the military a career and becoming an officer. Have you ever heard the saying, "When you want to make your creator laugh, tell Him your plans"? Well, my well-laid plans changed one day while working out at Randolph Air Force Base, San Antonio Texas.

During my work out this particular day, a gentleman approached me and asked me what did to get in such great shape. I told him jokingly, "I work out!" After speaking with him for a few minutes, I discovered he was a local celebrity bodybuilder. He was impressed with my physique and asked if I had ever thought about competing in a fitness competition.

At the time of our conversation, I wasn't familiar with such an event, therefore, a few days later I did some research into fitness competitions. I was excited about what I had learned. When I ran into the same gentleman a few weeks later at the gym, I told him that I thought I'd do great in a fitness competition and wanted to compete. He asked if he could train me for my first fitness show, and I agreed.

After agreeing to be trained by him, I began a rigorous fitness regimen, sometimes hitting the gym twice a day, six days per week! Eventually all of my hard work paid off. On May 12, 2001, after six months of this intense training, I stepped on stage for my first fitness competition. I remember being excited and nervous at the same time, but once I stepped on stage and the music began to play, I knew I was at home. I did amazing and took home first place and the overall fitness title. Needless to say, I found a new passion!

As time marched on and I continued to compete in fitness events, I eventually became one of the world's top ranked fitness competitors making it all the way to the Fitness Olympia where I was ranked eighth in the world in 2008. As my fitness career took off, more and more people began to ask me how I got into such great shape. At the time, I didn't know the anatomy and physiology behind my passion, but I knew I wanted to provide people with the tools to take control of their lives by getting healthier.

Therefore, in 2001, I decided to follow my passion, and I left the military on a mission to pursue my education in health. I went on the earn three degrees with my most recent one being a Master's Degree in Public Health and Public Administration. Along with my academic credentials, I have been featured in over 13 National and International Fitness, Health and Wellness Magazines, and I have also been featured as the go-to health and fitness expert for TV stations such as C.W. 31, Fox 45, ABC 22, Blab TV, WEAR 3, and many more.

It's Not about Me!

Although I am certainly grateful for all of my individual accomplishments, I am most grateful for all of the opportunities I have had to educate, empower and enhance the lives of adults and children through health and fitness. I have built my career on the saying, "People don't care how much you know until they know how much you care."

My greatest hope is to leave this world a healthier place. I have been blessed with the opportunity to work towards my goal, and I am determined to keep on working to build a legacy of healthy people. I've seen the damage that poor health wrecks on both communities and individuals, and if I can change someone's life one meal, one walk and one health seminar at a time, I will know my efforts were all worthwhile.

I honestly believe that when a person finds his or her passion that is the day he or she begins to live. I am forever grateful that I have found my passion, and I thank you for allowing me to share it with you!

Action Jackson~ "The Most Important Size a Woman Can Be is a Size Healthy"

Part 1
CHANGING THE NORM!

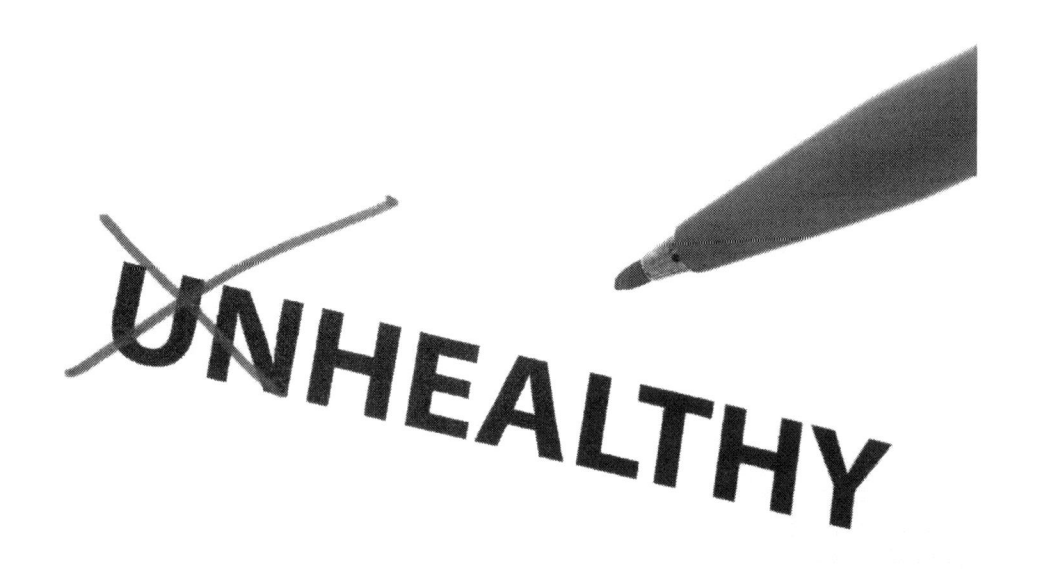

Chapter 1

Obesity, The Great Epidemic

If you watch the news, you will often hear about the great obesity epidemic that is plaguing millions of Americans. Research shows that 1/3 of U.S. adults are obese. What's even more alarming about this statistic is that obesity affects African Americans, especially African-American women at a disproportionate or higher rate than any other race.

According to the Centers for Disease Control (CDC), four out five African-American women are obese and are more likely to suffer from health conditions such as type 2 diabetes, cardiovascular disease, stroke, heart disease and some forms of cancer at higher rates than any other racial or ethnic group.

Why Such a Gap?

Why is there such a gap and why are African-American women more obese than any other race?

Great question!

First, allow me to say obesity is a multi-factored issue that can't be solved on an individualized level alone. It is individualized and systemic.

However as discussed in the introduction, the culture, and environment of many African-American women encourage and support the notion of "thickness" as the "NORM" and to change this alarming statistic, this notion has to be addressed first on an individual level!

Let's Have Sister Talk!

Before I go any further, I want to explain where I am coming from. My words are coming from a place of honesty and truth, and in my truth it is my hope that you will find empowerment to change what has always been accepted as the "NORM" or the normal way of living in our culture.

Your health is my priority. Therefore, I will share things with you that may seem uncomfortable to address, nonetheless, I will be honest and transparent with you about what has become the "NORM" and encourage you to see yourself and your health in a new perspective.

Now that you know that I have your best interest at heart, let's get back to addressing the notion of being "THICK."

Girl, I'm THICK!

From a genetic standpoint, African-American women's bodies are structured differently from other races or ethnicities. Due to our genetic structure we are more prone to carry excess body fat in our mid-sections and lower bodies which often gives us our "thick" appearance.

Carrying excess body fat in these areas make African-American women more prone to heart disease and other forms of cancer. What is very concerning is, too often we associate being "thick" as a good thing, when in all actuality it's killing us, and I will explain why!

What Is Obesity and How Is It Determined?

I've mentioned obesity, but what is obesity and how is it determined?

A person is classified or determined to be obese if their Body Mass Index (BMI) or the percentage of body fat is 30 percent or higher. We can go even further, a person is considered morbidly (greatly) obese if their BMI is 40 percent or higher.

Now that we have an understanding of the definition of obesity let's discuss how we gather the information that determines if one is obese or morbidly obese.

What is the Body Mass Index?

In the previous section, I mentioned Body Mass Index, and if you have never heard of this term before, you may be wondering what a Body Mass Index (BMI) is.

A Body Mass Index (BMI) is a number that is determined by using a person's height converted into inches then squared. Once this number is determined, it is divided by a person's weight converted into kilograms.

This mathematical equation can be done easily online by using a Body Mass Index Calculator (such as the one available at www.blackdoctors.org) or by using the Body Mass Index Chart, which you can locate below.

What is the Body Mass Index (BMI) Chart?

The Body Mass Index Chart is a suggested guideline for how much a person should weigh based on his or her height.

Some argue that the BMI scale isn't an accurate measurement tool for African-American women since it does not take into consideration lean muscle density and other factors that contribute to African-American women's Bodies. Although there's part truth to this statement, the BMI Scale is a good predictive tool for health conditions associated with individuals with a BMI of 30 percent or higher.

However, if you don't want to use the BMI Scale, a more accurate and dependable measure of body fat would be hydrostatic weighing or the weighing of one under the water. This tool is an effective body fat measuring tool; however, it has setbacks such as cost, participant's fear of water and limited access to weighing service.

From a convenience and accessibility standpoint, using the BMI Scale is a more appropriate and cost effective measuring tool.

Some hospital services such as weight management and dietetics can perform this service for you. You may even go to your local gym and have someone do your BMI for you at little to no cost.

It's Not That Simple!

Before I go any further, allow me to make this statement: Obesity is a complex issue that can't be fixed by just telling African-American women to exercise, eat healthier and maintain a healthy BMI.

Although research has proven consuming a healthy well-balanced diet, maintenance of a healthy body weight and regular physical activity can assist in the prevention of obesity, there are many other contributing factors on a system level that contribute to obesity.

These contributing factors include cultural barriers to health care, socioeconomics, perceived racism, poverty, health policies, food deserts (limited access to healthy foods), limited parks and safe areas for exercise, and a lack of transportation.

Each of these factors plays a key role in obesity within the African-American female population and will need to be addressed continually on a state and national level.

However, for the sake of this book we will discuss factors such as stress management, healthy nutrition, and regular physical activity that are more on an individual level that you can control. Let's get back to talking about obesity!

Is Obesity Costing You?

In addition to the health risks associated with obesity, obesity is expensive to treat and could be hindering your family's finances.

According to the Harvard School of Public Health, "By one estimate, the U.S. spent $190 billion on obesity-related health care expenses in 2005—double previous estimates" (Harvard, 2014).

In addition to this research the CDC estimates that the medical costs for people who are obese is $1,429 higher than those of normal weight (CDC, 2012).

Have you and your family felt the financial burden of your weight related illnesses?

Has taking medication for weight related issues such as type 2 diabetes and high blood pressure placed financial strain on you? If it has, take a moment to imagine the amount of money that can be saved to go towards other investments such as retirement, college tuition, family vacations, new cars and much more if a healthy body weight is maintained throughout your life span.

This definitely gives you something to think about, doesn't it?

Hard to Hear!

I know the conversation we are having is a hard one to have, but nonetheless it is a necessary one. Knowledge is only power when we expose the truth and then take action with the knowledge we have been given.

Do you agree?

CHANGING THE NORM

Let's Keep Moving Forward

By now it is my hope that you have a clearer understanding of obesity and realize that on a personal level there are things you can do to change your risk. We have only touched the surface in our sister talks.

Let's move forward and go a little deeper.

Are you ready?

Here we go!

Sister to Sister Tip: Creating a Healthy Body Weight Is Key To Improving Your Overall Health

Chapter 2

Is Your Confidence Killing You?

Allow me to ask you a question?

While you were reading the last chapter were you saying to yourself "I'm not obese and "I'm fine with my body weight?"

If you stated this and medically it has been proven you aren't obese this is great news. However, if you stated this, and you've been told by your doctor or other healthcare providers that you need to lose weight and you don't agree with what has been told to you, you are not alone. This statement is often echoed by many African-American women that I have had the honor and privilege of speaking to.

On one hand, it is amazing that we love our bodies; on the other hand, it is dangerous that we don't realize that our "NORM" and our body confidence may be killing us!

I Love My Body!

Having discussions about a woman's body and weight loss can be a very sensitive and often personal struggle for many women. However, one of the most interesting dynamics about obesity and African-American women is how we see our bodies and our body weight.

Numerous studies have shown that although African-American women have the highest rates of obesity, for many African-American women, the current state of their body weight isn't seen as a problem when compared to other races and ethnicities.

In the areas of self-confidence and body acceptance, research shows that African American women are ranked high in the areas of self-esteem and self-confidence.

As a person who advocates and empowers women to feel good about themselves, this is great news. However this great news also presents a great concern!

CHANGING THE NORM

I'm Fine the Way I Am!

Do you ever find yourself telling yourself that there's no need for you to change your body? What about, my man likes me the way that I am?

If this is you, I have to share a story with you that broke my heart.

But He Likes Me This Way!

One day while I was out shopping, a young lady approached me and asked what I did to get into such great shape. I responded to her question and shared with her my workout and healthy eating regimen.

As we continued our conversation, she began to say that she wanted and needed to lose weight, but she didn't do anything about it.

When I asked her why she didn't try to get healthier, she stated "My boyfriend doesn't want me to lose weight; he likes me 'THICK' and doesn't want me to get skinny."

This broke my heart!

I said to her in a very loving manner, "You getting healthy isn't about what he wants, it's what you need and deserve!"

This young African-American woman had bought into the "NORM" that black men love their women "THICK" and she was willing to place a man's needs above her own.

Where am I going with this?

If you have the opportunity to get healthier, why not invest in yourself?

Yes, you're beautiful, smart, fine, curvy, and even sexy, but are you allowing what someone else wants and desires to put your health at risk?

This is a question that every African-American woman needs to ask herself!

I understand the struggle of wanting to be pleasing to your spouse or significant other, but I would like to assume that you getting healthy will allow him to see you in a different but positive light.

Remember, you don't have to get rid of your curves to be healthy! Getting healthier isn't about you becoming a size small, it's about you becoming a size healthy!

Therefore apply these 5 simple tips to start focusing more on your health:

5 Tips to Start Focusing on Your Health

1) **Be Honest With Yourself:** Being honest with yourself about the condition of your body is essential if you're going to get healthier. If you haven't been good to your body, it's acceptable to acknowledge this to yourself. Saying it out loud will allow you to take ownership of your role. This isn't a time for condemnation, just acknowledgment.

2) **Apply the Rule of 7:** Commit to doing 1 healthy thing per day and by the end of the week you have done 7 healthy things for yourself. I call this my Rule of 7 Principle. This principle is simple and creates a daily awareness of your food and physical activity choices.

3) **Just Move!:** Commit to moving your body by walking or exercising 3-5 days per week for at least 30 minutes per day. Research from The American College of Sports Medicine (ACSM) has shown that exercising at least 30 minutes 5 days per week can yield great health benefits.

   If you can't walk 5 days per week, start off slow and aim for at least 2-3 days per week. If you don't live in a safe area where you can walk at a park or in your neighborhood, find somewhere safe and walk indoors in places such as a mall or a shopping center.

4) **Refuse to Buy a Larger Size:** Buying larger sized clothes can give you a reason not to be mindful of your weight gain. Therefore, if you notice yourself gaining weight, REFUSE to buy any clothes that are a larger size. Instead, focus on your eating and physical activities as a way to combat your weight gain.

5) **Make a Commitment:** Making a commitment to your health is one of the best decisions you can make for yourself and those who love you. When you make a commitment to your health, you're telling the world and yourself that you are WORTH the time, money and energy required to take care of yourself!

It is essential that I tell you that getting healthy isn't an easy process. Nonetheless it is a process that has to start somewhere.

CHANGING THE NORM

Therefore REFUSE to spend another day allowing yourself or anyone else to stop you from reaching a better state of health.

The world needs you, but more important, you need you!

Sister To Sister Tip: It Is Essential To Make Yourself a Priority in Your Life, By Doing So, You Can Create More Time For Your Health

Chapter 3

Why Can't You Change?

In the previous chapter, we talked about how your environment can hinder the change process and you were provided with 5 tips to assist you in focusing more on your health.

Now it's time to discover why changing your lifestyle will be a challenge even after you've made the decision to get healthy.

Change is a Process!

We are often told by our physicians, healthcare providers, and, sometimes our significant others or loved ones that we need to get healthier, but we are seldom given direction on how to get started.

We are lead to believe that the only thing required to change is to make the decision to do so and motivation. This assumption is far from the truth and what can be even more discouraging is that once you have made the decision to change, you start off with great excitement and zeal and then you hit a wall and lose your desire to keep going.

Can you say frustrating?

Have you ever experienced this?

We've all been there and it goes a little something like this.

This Time, I'm Going To Do It!

You surf the internet or finally seek out help to get you started in the right direction. This help could come in the form of a personal trainer or health coach.

You clean out your refrigerator, buy new exercise equipment and workout clothes.

For about a month or two you're fully committed to getting healthier, but seemingly and all of a sudden you just can't stick with it.

In your mind you know what you need to do. However, you just can't change your unhealthy behaviors!

CHANGING THE NORM

My friend, allow me to say this is normal and what you're experiencing is known as the stages of change.

Yes, change has stages. Allow me to explain the five stages of behavior change and why changing can be a very hard to accomplish.

Stages of Change What?

Over the years, I have sat with hundreds of frustrated individuals who want to change but don't understand why changing their behaviors is such a challenge.

As one can imagine, not having a "WHY" can be discouraging and often a barrier to becoming healthier.

To help you avoid or discontinue feeling this way, I will provide you with the 5 stages that occur when someone considers changing their behaviors.

If you have a journal, I recommend you take notes.

What are the Stages of Change?

The five stages of change include: Pre-Contemplation, Contemplation, Preparation, Action, and Maintenance. We will also discuss a possible stage known as the relapse stage.

Let's discuss what occurs during each stage of change.

1) **Pre-Contemplation:** In this stage of change, a person doesn't recognize that she needs to make a change and doesn't plan on doing anything different within the next 6 months, regardless of what she hears from others.

    The individual in this stage of change often ignores or denies their current condition (example: Someone tells Alice that it would be beneficial to her health if she started walking to shed some unhealthy weight. She gets up and walks away and says, "My weight is fine just the way it is.").

2) **Contemplation:** In this stage of change, an individual begins to think about making a change within the next 6 months and begins to weigh the pros of making a change (**example:** If I start eating healthier I could possibly lose weight and be taken off of my blood pressure medication).

3) **Preparation:** In this stage of change, an individual begins to make the necessary plans to begin their process of change (example: Sally went to her community YMCA and signed up for their group fitness class.)

4) **Action:** In this stage of change, an individual is actively doing the things that she needs to do to reach her desired goal (example: Sally has been eating small healthy meals every 2-3 hours and she's logging all of her meals in her meal planner for the last 2 months).

5) **Maintenance:** In this stage of change, a person is maintaining their new behaviors and is less apt to go back to their old lifestyle behaviors. (example: Sally has been eating healthy, working out and getting at least 8 hours of sleep per night for over 6 months. She feels and looks great.) The longer a person remains in the stage of change the less likely they will revert to old lifestyle behaviors.

*Possible Stage of Change

Relapse: In this stage of change a person goes back to their old behaviors. This is often triggered by stress or unsupportive environments. If or when a person goes back to old behaviors it is essential to identify the triggers and determine new coping mechanisms and support systems to deal accordingly.

Now that wasn't too bad was it?

That may have seemed to be a lot of information, but keep in mind, you're learning new information and it doesn't mean that you have to understand or apply all of the information your learning at one time.

Change Doesn't Happen Overnight!

Although we have discussed the stages of change, I want you to understand that the changes you desire to make won't happen overnight.

I know with all the commercials you see promising your drastic weight loss with the popping of a few pills and no diet exercise, it is easy to believe in instantaneous changes.

These commercials are misleading and the inventors of these products are making millions of dollars per year. However the rate of obesity continues to affect African-American women therefore, I'd like to encourage you to refrain from buying into the get fit or lose quick philosophy. It doesn't WORK!

CHANGING THE NORM

Once again, allow me to re-emphasize that permanent weight loss is a result of making behavior or lifestyle changes over a period of time and does not and will not occur overnight with diet pills or get fit quick fixes!

Besides, you're way too smart to accept this "NORM"!

Slow Down and Breathe!

As you engage in the change process, remember behavior change isn't about correcting all of your unhealthy behaviors at once. Rather, it's about first making the commitment to yourself to get healthier one behavior at a time.

While you're on your way to making one healthy behavior change at a time, set realistic short-term goals and reward yourself with non-food items when you set and meet a goal.

Most importantly, believe you are worth the money, time, and effort that will be required of you to make a lifestyle change.

Remember that I am right here cheering you on all the way.

Can you hear me shouting your name?

What's Your Motivation?

I am guessing you probably didn't think you were going to get so much information in one place did you?

I've decided to provide you with so much information based on the fact that I believe in that old cliché that states "If you give a man a fish, he eats for a day. If you TEACH a man to fish and he eats for a lifetime.

I am teaching you how to get healthy for a lifetime! Pretty awesome right?

Let's take a breather for just a moment and have what I call a brain break. Okay, did you rest your brain for a second?

Great!

Let's keep moving forward and discuss motivation!

Chapter 4

What's Your Motivation?

We're about to talk about motivation! You know that word so many people believe they lack?

Is It Motivation or Commitment?

Follow me down motivation lane if you will!

Has this ever happened to you?

You're excited about the new you and you're telling everyone about it. You've started your new workout program, eating healthy, and you have even bought some new clothes to show off your new body!

You're 100 percent committed for about a month because you have got to get your fine on to get into that dress for your friend's wedding or you've got to get into that swimsuit for the summer.

You work out faithfully and no one better touch your healthy foods. You make it to your event and all of a sudden you exhale and can't wait to get back to your old way of doing things!

Does this sound all too familiar to you?

If you have tried to get healthier in the past and only reached a certain point, you may believe you lack motivation and that's the reason you haven't been successful.

I'd like to challenge you to re-think your thought process.

A lack of motivation alone may not be the problem or the reason why you haven't reached your goals and stayed consistent with maintaining healthy behaviors.

Your lack of follow through may be due to a lack of commitment.

Yes, a lack of commitment. Stay with me and don't tune me out.

Are you with me?

Great, let's move on.

CHANGING THE NORM

Here's the Problem with Motivation!

Here's the problem with motivation.

I know this sounds contradictory, but I'm going somewhere with this.

Motivation is often brought on by an emotion and once that particular emotion has left, motivation is thrown out the door like a week old gallon of milk.

You know that feeling of wanting to fit back into that favorite black dress or your desire to look really great at your 20-year class reunion?

You're so motivated to reach your goal that you commit to the gym seven days a week.

You get up early to get to the gym, you pack your healthy foods before leaving home and you're in bed at a decent time.

Sounds like a great plan of action doesn't it?

It is, but here's where motivation gets us all in trouble when we aren't committed to long-term healthy living.

Once you've reached your short-term goal, the motivation to eat healthy and exercise on a regular basis is over! You exhale and go back to your normal way of living, and when you venture back to your old lifestyle behaviors you typically bring a few extra unwanted pounds along with you.

I see you smiling and I hear you laughing out loud! This has happened to you before hasn't it?

Come on, be honest, we are all guilty of doing this at least once -- alright, twice -- in our lifetimes.

Since we are all guilty of such behavior, how can we avoid this lack of commitment trap?

Avoid the Commitment Trap

The first step to avoiding the commitment trap is to make the decision to get fit and healthy for more than aesthetic or superficial reasons.

There's nothing wrong with desiring to look good in your clothing!

However, if you attach long-term value such as a better quality of life, better mobility (movement) to play with your children, or the ability to experience better overall health, you have a better chance of staying committed.

CHANGING THE NORM

The second step is to not rely on your emotions to determine whether or not you should do something healthy.

Emotions are so untrustworthy. When you look great, you desire to stick to the healthy path you're on. When the scale is dropping and pounds are shedding, your emotions are high, but when the numbers go up on the scale, your emotions are low.

You get where I am going.

Don't trust your emotions; rather, trust your commitment.

Trust your commitment to yourself, that, regardless of how long it takes you to reach your health and fitness goals, you are committed to your health for the long haul.

This means when you don't feel like going to the gym because that old swimsuit or dress didn't fit when you tried it on, you still go.

It means eating healthy when you can have fast food even when the scale hasn't gone down all week.

A commitment to yourself is a commitment to yourself; regardless of what your emotions tell you.

Therefore, before we move on to the next chapter I want you to think about your top five reasons for wanting to get healthier.

I also want you to think about the top three challenges you may face in regards to reaching your desired destination.

Discovering the answers to these questions will provide you with the **"Why"** to what you are about to embark on.

Don't rush yourself to answer these questions; take the time to reflect and be honest about your commitment to your health journey.

_____
_____
_____
_____
_____

Chapter 5

Remove the Mask

In the previous chapter I encouraged you to determine your commitment to your health, now I want to address factors that could influence the amount of time and effort you commit to yourself.

I Got This!

It is no secret that Black Women often carry their communities, families and careers on their shoulders.

We're mothers, wives, CEOs, Pastors and the list goes on. Unfortunately, we have been so busy carrying the entire world around on our shoulders that we have forgotten how to take care of ourselves and far too many of us have bought into that potentially hazardous notion that says, "I'm a STRONG Black woman, I GOT this!"

You've said this before haven't you?

If we're honest, we have all said this before!

Here's where we have allowed this strong statement to affect our health and we have to change this "NORM".

I'm a STRONG Black Woman

Because we are "STRONG BLACK WOMEN", many of us seldom ask for help when it's needed.

Instead of saying we need help or desire help, we take many burdens and responsibilities upon ourselves and day after day, we carry stress in our bodies.

We seldom make time for exercise; proper eating and most importantly, we don't make time to de-stress.

In essence, we put our "I GOT THIS" mask on and tell the entire world that we're just fine!

I've done it, and I suspect it's safe to say that you've done this very thing at times as well.

Remember we're having sister talk here and there's no need to feel ashamed.

CHANGING THE NORM

We can't change the "NORM" if we aren't willing to acknowledge our truth!

So often we hold strong to the belief that, "I'm a STRONG BLACK WOMAN" until we find ourselves, overworked, overwhelmed and often overweight!

Is this you?

If it is, it's time to REMOVE your mask and learn to ask for help to make more time for yourself and your health.

Asking for help isn't a sign of weakness, rather a sign of strength. There's strength in the ability to acknowledge that you need someone else to help you on your journey.

Therefore, it's time to step away from your mask; you are no longer auditioning for a play.

Will the real you stand up?

The Audition is Over

Removing the masks you've worn for so long can be a difficult process, yet it is necessary to reveal a true reflection of yourself.

Deciding to let go of old facades can result in many personal challenges and cause you to look deep within yourself and challenge many of your long-held beliefs and coping mechanisms.

Yes, coping mechanisms. We all have them and food may be the one that keeps you safe from all of the storms in your life!

Addressing these challenges may not be easy, but, in the long run, it will be worth it.

It's time to set yourself free, you need YOU!

Stranger in the Midst

So where do you go from here?

It sounds great to remove the masks you've worn for so long, but once you have removed your masks and discover you're not content with what you find, how do you move forward?

Besides, years have gone by and you may have gotten married, changed jobs, given birth or completed your education.

CHANGING THE NORM

You're grateful for your life and excited about your accomplishments, but you've discovered that you're not happy with how you have let yourself go.

You're exhausted, your body's turning against you, and in many ways feel like you've lost yourself.

Just Exhale

First things, first. Slow down, exhale and realize that it's never too late to change.

If you're starting to feel bad, there's no need to beat yourself up.

However it is time to say goodbye to your Superwoman Cape and MOVE forward.

Superwoman Isn't Your Name

If you have ever felt the need to shout, "I need time to myself," welcome to the Superwoman Club!

As women, we often find ourselves taking care of others as if it is programmed into our DNA and too often we believe that saying "no" is a cardinal sin.

You know exactly what I am talking about don't you?

If you do, lean in for a moment and allow me tell you a little secret, come a little closer.

Are you leaning in?

Great!

I want to tell you that it is perfectly acceptable to take off your Superwoman cape for 30 minutes at least three days per week to do something healthy for yourself. If you don't take care of yourself, how can you take care of anyone else?

Let me ask you a few questions!

When was the last time you made time for yourself?

Do you often tell yourself that someday you will get back to you?

If you've been saying someday, that someday is now!

Today is the day to start afresh!

It's time to recommit to you!

It's Time to Commit to Yourself!

Making a renewed commitment to yourself doesn't mean you have to look like the fitness models in the magazines, but it is possible to create a new and improved version of yourself.

Whatever your goal may be you have to create action steps to get there!

How do you accomplish this?

Get Back on Track

The first step to getting back on track is to acknowledge what you do not like about yourself!

This may sound contradictory to the message of this book. However it's an essential part of the self-reflection process.

Remember we can't change what we don't acknowledge!

Once this task has been completed, ask yourself on a scale of 0-10 (0 low- 10 high) how willing, able and confident you are to address these issues.

From there, determine the steps needed to make your desired changes. Be patient and kind with yourself and realize it will take time to make a change.

Second, establish a support system and communicate your needs and challenges. Sometimes making a change requires guidance and support.

If you have gained weight and need further assistance to get you on the right track, review your budget to see if you can afford a personal trainer or gym membership.

If this isn't feasible, there are several options such as community recreation centers or churches that offer free fitness programs.

If you can't fit a trainer into your budget, you can purchase or rent fitness videos for home. You may also workout at the park or go for regular walks around your neighborhood if you reside in a safe area.

To allow greater support, encourage your husband/significant other to help around the house to free up more time for yourself and if time permits, create a fitness regimen for the both of you. This will provide one-on-one time to build teamwork and spend valuable time together.

Need new healthy food ideas; this book is full of them.

Lastly, and most importantly, believe you have the ability to change whatever it is that you don't like about yourself.

If you know that you haven't devoted enough time to your health, acknowledge this and move forward.

Don't get stuck in a place of should have's and would have's. This is negative and unproductive!

Believing in yourself will give you the motivation to keep going when times become rough.

Don't Allow Age To Stop You

As you are making changes, I want to forewarn you that your mind will attempt to create reasons as to why you can't change. Age may become one of those false reasons.

I've experienced this way too many times not to warn you. Unfortunately, I often hear, "I'm too old to be exercising." When in all actuality, regardless of your age, if you have a heart beat you should be moving! That means EVERYONE despite their age needs to move and become healthy!

Has Age Stopped You?

What about you? Have you allowed your age to be a barrier to you getting healthier?

For many women, age has become a logical reason as to why they aren't getting into shape.

The media is popular for subliminally telling women that when they reach a certain age, it's all downhill from there.

This is far from the truth!

If you feel this way, you need to know age literally is just a number. There's no denying that as women age it's harder for them to get into shape, but it's not impossible.

Do not allow this mentality to prevent you from reaching your health and fitness goals.

It's NEVER too Late!

If you feel it is too late, meet Sandra.

At the age of forty-eight, Sandra weighed over 200 pounds at 5"4". She was isolated and not living a very adventurous life.

After a regular visit to her doctor, she realized she was sick and tired of being sick and tired and that it was time to do something about her health.

To start making changes towards her health, she began making small steps, such as making healthier food choices. Then, she eventually began incorporating regular exercise into her everyday routine.

When Sandra and I met, she was ready to begin her new fitness journey, and as her personal trainer, I was able to guide and assist her in reaching her fitness and various health goals.

When Sandra came to me, she brought focus, dedication and commitment to her new lifestyle. She made my job as her trainer an inspiring experience.

Her dedication and commitment to her health allowed her to go from weighing over 200 pounds to weighing 154 pounds 6 months later. In November 2010, she ran her first 5k and continues to set new health and fitness goals. I have stayed in contact with Sandra and she like many women often finds it difficult to stay on track with healthy living.

Nonetheless, she's committed to her health, and when she falls from the health and fitness wagon, she has already made up in her mind that she's going to continue to get back up and move forward.

Sandra recently celebrated her 53 birthday and her new life is the best present she could have given herself.

Every time I see her, I am inspired by her transformation and honored to be a part of her health and fitness journey.

Just like Sandra, you too can reach your health and fitness goals!

Embrace Your Age!

Embrace your age and view it as an asset and not a liability. Your age won't stop you from reaching your goals, but a lack of commitment and follow-through will.

I have no doubt in my mind that you can do this and if your age is preventing you from moving forward, refuse to be held hostage by a number.

Use these following tips to help you succeed on your health and fitness journey!

Prepare to Succeed

Getting fit at any age can be a challenge, but planning for your fitness success can assist you in reaching your desired destination.

Let me show you how to get on board and stay on board with your fitness goals at an older age.

- ✓ Make a list of challenges that are keeping you from setting and reaching your fitness and health goals. Be honest and make realistic goals to change these behaviors. Take one-step at a time to change these behaviors. Be patient: change will not occur overnight.
- ✓ Surround yourself with other women in your age group who are dedicated to getting fit. Forming a strong support system is essential to your success and will provide you with support from other women who may experience the same emotional and physical challenges.
- ✓ As you reach your goals, reward yourself with non-food items to celebrate your success. Possibly get a new dress, shoes or purse. Make it special and to your likings. Maybe book yourself to see your favorite R& B artist.
- ✓ Share your accomplishments with individuals in your support system who love you and believe in you. They won't downplay your success and they will know how hard you have worked to get there.
- ✓ Continue to hold yourself accountable for making progress and don't allow your age to be a barrier to reaching your fitness goals. In order to do this, find an accountability partner to help you stay consistent and dedicated. If you find yourself discouraged, address the causes of your discouragement and move forward.
- ✓ If you fall off track, do not beat yourself up. Get back up, brush the dust off and move forward with your fitness goals. Everyone gets sidetracked every now and then.

- ✓ If you become bored with your fitness goals, set new ones. This will keep you engaged and excited about your fitness program and reaching your desired fitness destination.
- ✓ Take your workouts to the pool. As we age, we may experience arthritis and other joint problems. If you experience joint problems with physical activities, take your exercise to the pool. Exercising in the water places less stress on the joints and allows more pain-free movements.

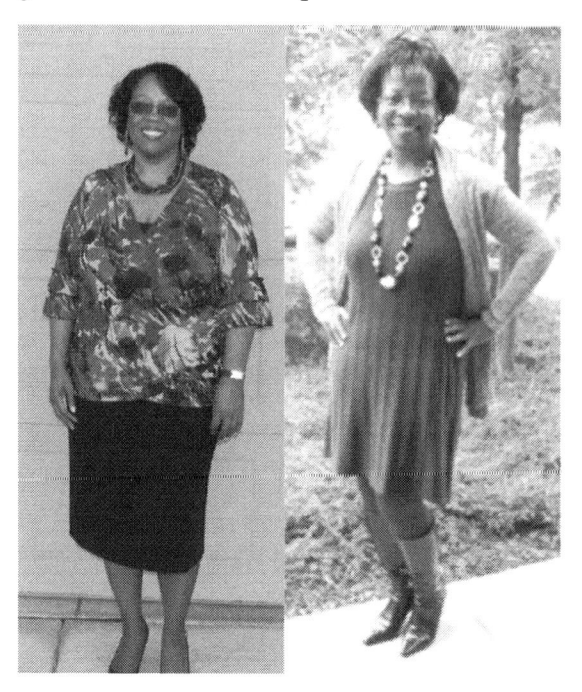

Before	After
April 2009	October
219 lbs	150 lbs

Chapter 6

A Heart Beat Away

A part of loving yourself is to learn about the health issues that affect you as a woman, especially as an African American woman. As we discussed earlier, it is important to take more time for your health. In doing so, I want to talk about the number one killer of women. That number one killer is heart disease.

Heart disease affects millions of women annually, but this life-threatening condition affects African-American women at higher rates than any other race or ethnicity. Let's look at some very alarming statistics!

Statistics from the American Heart Association are alarming!
- ✓ Cardiovascular diseases kill nearly 50,000 African-American women annually.
- ✓ Of African-American women ages 20 and older, 49 percent have heart diseases.
- ✓ Only one in five African-American women believes she is personally at risk.
- ✓ Only 52 percent of African-American women are aware of the signs and symptoms of a heart attack.
- ✓ Only 36 percent of African-American women know that heart disease is their greatest health risk.

Were you aware of these alarming statistics?

Did you know this many African-American women die each year from heart disease?

Has anyone you know died from heart disease?

There's Truth in the Numbers

Did providing you with these statistics from the American Heart Association provide you with better insight as to why you have to TAKE time for your health?

As I mentioned at the beginning of this book, if we are going to change the "NORM" we must acknowledge where we are with our health and continue to make strides together in improving how we take care of our bodies.

Do you agree?

If you do, let's have more HEART talk about why it is so important to keep the heart healthy.

Why is your heart health more important than a six-pack?

The heart is the body's main engine that provides oxygen-rich blood to all functioning organs, tissues and bones.

Unhealthy lifestyle behaviors from smoking, a lack of physical activity, poor dietary choices and chronic stress can contribute to heart disease and place African-American women at risk for stroke which is the 3rd leading cause of death for Americans.

Heart disease is preventable in most cases however, one of the major concerns regarding heart disease is that many African-American women have heart disease and don't know they have it.

In all honesty, you could be seconds away from having a heart attack.

It happens every day!

How Does Heart Disease Happen?

Yes, you may be seconds away from having a heart attack!

I know this is something you don't want to hear, but it's something that you need to hear.

Therefore allow me to explain how a heart attack happens!

You're Just a Second Away!

The heart is a strong muscle that pumps without being told (involuntary) many times during the day. When your heart pumps, it uses arteries to carry nutrients and oxygen-rich blood to your entire body. This flow of blood is stopped or hindered when your arteries become clogged as a result of unhealthy living.

CHANGING THE NORM

A Picture is Worth a Million Words

After years of unhealthy living, the inside lining of your blood vessels become covered with a white substance called cholesterol or plague. Over time, this plaque can become hardened and can potentially stop the blood flow to your heart or brain resulting in a heart attack or stroke (the third ranking killer of Americans). This hardening process is known as atherosclerosis or the hardening of your arteries.

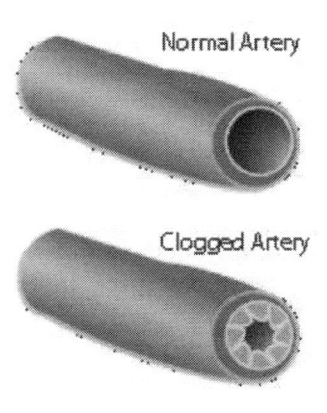

Normal Artery

Clogged Artery

How can you prevent this from happening?

There are many ways, let's discuss a few!

Do You Know Your Numbers?

The image shown above may not have been what you were looking for; however, I am here to teach you the dangers associated with an unhealthy lifestyle.

Heart disease is a real concern for African-American women and I refuse not do my part. My part is to inform and educate you on the severity of this disease and provide you with the knowledge that heart disease can be prevented!

Therefore allow me to provide you with a few things you can do take lessen your risk of heart disease.

Lessen Your Risk

The first way to lessen your risk or of heart disease is to know your blood pressure numbers, cholesterol readings and family history of heart disease.

Your blood pressure and cholesterol readings can both be done by your doctor or healthcare provider such as a Nurse Practitioner and should be taken annually or more often based on your health condition.

If you don't have access to your own doctor, a community health department in your area should offer these tests for free or at a minimal cost.

It is essential to emphasize that knowing these numbers could help save your life!

In addition to knowing your blood pressure and cholesterol levels, it is important to know your family history.

Genetics play a major role in your health conditions; therefore ask around to determine if anyone in your family has a history of heart disease. If your parents are still living, it is essential to speak with them about heart disease. If either of your parents have heart disease, you're more at risk.

The second way to lessen your risk of heart disease is to know the signs of a heart attack.

Heart attacks displays itself differently in women compared to men, therefore, become heart healthy and learn the signs and symptoms of heart disease for women (see symptoms listed below).

The third step you can take to lessen your risk of heart disease is to stop smoking, eat healthier and exercise on a regular basis.

Research has shown that weight reduction, healthy eating, and not smoking can lessen your risk of heart disease.

Symptoms of Heart Disease

For many years, heart disease was considered a man's disease and due to this old belief, many women were left in the dark about their risk for heart disease. Unfortunately, this resulted in thousands of women being undiagnosed.

Today there's an abundance of research on how to prevent, identify and treat heart disease. This information has helped saved lives of women of identified to have heart disease.

Do You Know the Signs?

As with any disease, early prevention and detection can assist in saving your life. Therefore, lets discover a few signs and symptoms of heart disease and heart attacks.

Symptoms of heart disease and heart attacks include but are not limited to nausea, back pain, shortness of breath, and sharp pain in the left side of the arm and dull or sharp pain in the chest (angina).

If you experience any of these symptoms, seek medical attention immediately and don't attribute it to something else. It is better to be sure than to guess.

Unfortunately, I have heard of too many cases where a woman had a heart attack or had heart disease but thought it was possibly gas or gastric issues.

Remember, it is always best to play it safe! Get to your doctor today and learn your numbers!

Do you know your numbers? If you don't, make an appointment with your physician today. Your heart can't wait any longer.

Total Cholesterol: <200 mg/dL
LDL "Bad" Cholesterol: **Optimal: <100 mg/dL**   **Near optimal/Above Optimal: 100-129 mg/dL**   **Borderline High: 130-159 mg/dL**   **High: 160-189 mg/dL**   **Very High: 190 mg/dL and above**
HDL ("Good") Cholesterol: 50 mg/dL or higher   **Triglycerides: <150 mg/dL**   **Blood Pressure: <120/80 mmHg**   **Fasting Glucose: <100 mg/dL**   **Body Mass Index: <25**   **Waist Circumference: <35 inches**

CHANGING THE NORM

For more information on women and heart disease log on to the following websites.

American Heart Association

www.americanheart.org

National Heart, Lung & Blood Institute

www.nhlbi.nih.gov

Chapter 7
Change Your Mind, Change Your Body

How's Your Thought Life?

In the last chapter a great amount of emphasis was placed on the functioning of your heart and how to prevent heart disease and heart attacks.

As we move forward, I'd like to now discuss another powerful part of your body. Your mind! Yes, your mind!

May I ask you a question?

Do you believe the current state of your body or health is the by-product or the result of you thought patterns?

Do you cringe at the thought of exercise and healthy eating?

Were you told as a child you were unattractive, not smart of good enough?

Have you accepted the notion that everyone in your family is overweight therefore it's fine to be overweight?

I know these aren't questions you want to be asked, however, I am my sister's keeper and as a sister, I love you enough to be honest with you! Your past can affect how you see your body and yourself.

Therefore, if your thoughts are holding you back, I want you to realize your thoughts can lead you down the road of fitness and weight loss success or your thoughts can lead you down the dead-end road of unhealthy and unhappy.

Which road will you choose?

Think Successful and Healthy Thoughts!

Allow me to share how important your thoughts about yourself really are!

I will use myself as an example!

Once I made the decision to become a professional athlete, I realized how important my thoughts would be to the success of my career.

The physical demands of training, injuries, the cost of competing, the struggle of being a full-time student, and family issues could have hindered me from reaching my goals if I allowed my thoughts to be thoughts of defeat.

Therefore, I realized early in my career that my level of success heavily depended upon my thoughts. Not just in my professional life, but also in my personal life.

This truth holds the same for you and reaching your health and fitness goals.

During moments of physical and mental fatigue, I would speak words of affirmation about myself to myself.

When negative thoughts crossed my mind, I would quickly replace them with positive ones. I am fully aware that years of negative thinking take time to address and develop new thought patterns. However, the first step in making progress is to address the negative thoughts that influence our behaviors.

On your personal health journey, you will have to create your own positive thoughts to help you reach your destination. If you discover deep rooted issues from your past, it's beneficial to seek out qualified counseling to assist you in understanding your internal thoughts.

At all times it is essential to remember, the power of life and death are in YOUR tongue.

That's right!

YOU have the power to change what you don't like!

Are you ready to change the conversations you have been having with yourself?

Take Control of Your Thoughts

Years ago I decided to create positive thoughts that would assist me in reaching my goals in life. As a result, I created my 3 D's of success.

My 3 D's of success created a road map for thinking that allowed me to challenge my thought life and assisted me in accomplishing many of my goals.

Therefore, I want to share my 3 D's of success with you. Use my 3 D's or create your own.

Your thoughts will always your compass in life! Therefore choose your thoughts wisely!

CHANGING THE NORM

The First D Is For Desire.

What do you desire?

1. The First D is for Desire

Whatever you desire, it has to be motivating enough to cause you to create and take the necessary steps to reach your destination. Desire has to be internal and it is something that doesn't have to be explained to anyone. Your desire has to be great enough to provoke a change within yourself and no one else.

- Do you desire to run and play with your children without getting tired?
- Do you desire to look at yourself in the mirror unclothed and like what you see?
- Do you desire to be more intimate with your husband and feel great about yourself?
- Do you desire to get off blood pressure medication?

2. The Second D Is For Discipline.

Discipline is Essential for Change!

Many of us do not like the word discipline, as it conveys hard work.

However, discipline is something you must possess to reach your desired goal(s).

It may mean getting up an hour earlier to get to the gym, or it could mean telling your closest friends that you can't hang out all night because you need eight hours of sleep to have an effective fitness training session the next day.

Whatever it may take, if you lack discipline, it will be hard to reach your fitness and health destination.

Therefore ask yourself are you willing to practice discipline on a consistent basis to reach your desired goal. The answer to this question will help you determine your current level of commitment to your health!

3. The Last D Stands For Determination.

Determination is something I hold very dear to my heart. There have been many times in life where chaos has threatened to take control.

During these moments, I had to make the choice to stay determined to reach my goals. It is essential to remember that chaos in your life does not constitute a reason to stop working towards your goals. Make the choice to work around your obstacles and refuse to accept "NO" for an answer!

Life Can Be OVERWHELMING!

The process of learning to change your thoughts will be a hard process; however, if you're dedicated to embracing this process, changing your thoughts can result in personal growth and development.

I will warn you in advance. There will be days when you want to throw in the towel and revert to negative ways of thinking. Therefore, when these moments happen, work hard to replace your negative thoughts with positive and reaffirming thoughts.

To help you become more successful during your change process, use the following tips.

- ✓ **Block the Thoughts:** You can't stop every negative thought from coming into your mind, but you can block many of them. Therefore when you or someone else begins to say negative things about you, stop them and yourself. Be kind but replace the negativity with something positive!
- ✓ **Have a Plan:** Write down your goals and the steps required to reach them. Having a visual plan and a frame of reference can help you get excited about your goals. Create a vision board and place it somewhere visible.
- ✓ **Share with the RIGHT people:** Only share your goals with people who believe in you and want to support you. Having negative people in your life is toxic and unproductive.
- ✓ **Take Baby Steps:** Take baby steps until you reach your destination. Don't get overwhelmed with the destination, instead focus on the journey. By doing this, you will feel less pressure and stress to reach your

goals. Remember it's a process. Celebrate your decision to get healthy and keep moving!

- ✓ **Celebrate Yourself:** Be proud of the progress you are making, whether big or small. Don't wait until you reach your big goal(s) before you celebrate. Every day that you move in a positive direction towards your goal is a day to be celebrated.
- ✓ **Be Gentle:** Be gentle and don't beat yourself up if you don't reach your goals by the deadline you've set. It's not a failure on our part. Sometimes we set unrealistic goals within an unrealistic period of time. When this happens, re-evaluate your goals and set more realistic ones in a more reasonable time frame.

Sister To Sister Tip: Creating New Thought Patterns About How Your See Yourself and Your Body Can Be A Challenging Yet Rewarding Process

Chapter 8

10 Days Of Inner Discovery

Seek and You Shall Find

The only items required for this section is a pen and an open heart!

Before you begin journaling find a quiet place where you can process your thoughts and emotions without being interrupted.

Being alone with yourself will provide you with the time needed to answer the following questions. As you move forward with this process, it is essential to understand that participating in Ten Days of Inner Discovery will require you to be honest with yourself about your past and the person you have become.

As you journal, I'd encourage you to be open to exploring areas within yourself that you may have been hidden away.

Discovering answers to hard asked questions may lead you down a path of emotional healing and freedom.

Often our body image and self-esteem are a reflection of our past experiences. By acknowledging and dealing with pain past experiences we can potentially assist you in moving forward with your life.

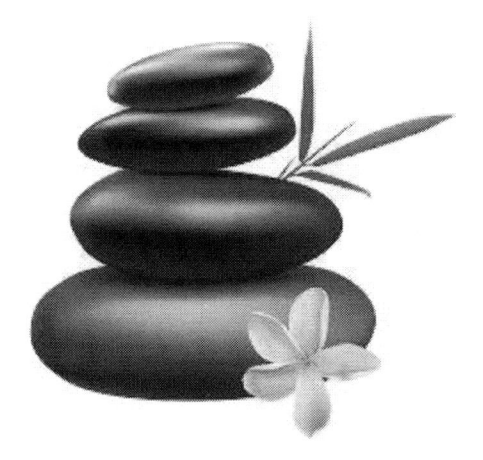

Seek and Ye Shall Find

Day 1

Today, you are going to take 15 to 20 minutes to reflect on your childhood experiences and write about them. Can you recall certain defining moments in your childhood? Were these moments happy or sad? Many of our behaviors and attitudes including our body image are shaped by our childhood experiences.

Take your time and don't be afraid to dive deep into your past.

Day 1 Journal Entry

Date:

Day 2: External Exploration

Write down all the physical things you do not like about yourself. Yes, I said that correctly - you are going to write down all the physical things you do not like about yourself. You probably have a puzzled look on your face. Stay with me; by the end of Day 10 you will completely understand.

Day 2 Journal Entry	Date:

Day 3: Mirror, Mirror on the Wall

Write down all the things you love about yourself. This task will be difficult for some and easy for others. If in your past people criticized you and told you that you were worthless, then you may have a hard time finding the good things within. However, dig deep and write down at least five things you love about yourself.

Day 3 Journal Entry

Date:

Day 4: Internal Revelation

Today's assignment is going to be thought-provoking. Make sure you have at least 15 to 20 minutes to write in your journal. Answer the following questions.

Day 4 Journal Entry Date:

1. Do you place everyone else needs above your own?

2. Do you feel overwhelmed with life but never ask for help? If yes, why?

3. Have you allowed the notion that you're a "Strong Black Woman" keep you from asking for help when needed?

4. Do you allow others opinions of you dictate how you see yourself?

5. Are you truly happy with your life?

6. Are past hurts keeping you from moving forward?

7. Do you believe life has a great plan for you?

8. Do you look at other people's lives and envy them?

9. Do you believe you can accomplish whatever you put your mind to?

10. Do you try new things or are you stuck in a rut?

11. Is your self-worth based on other people's opinion of you?

12. Do you seek happiness in money or material things?

Day 5: Today Is Dedicated To Pure Relaxation

Find a special place where no one else is allowed. Burn an aromatherapy candle, play some soft music and set the lights dimly. It may sound like you are preparing a place for a romantic dinner with someone else, but you are actually preparing for a special moment with yourself. Take 15 minutes to pray or meditate on your day. Do not feel bad; the earth will continue to rotate without you being there to turn it on its axis.

Meditation and relaxation have been shown to improve blood pressure and overall health

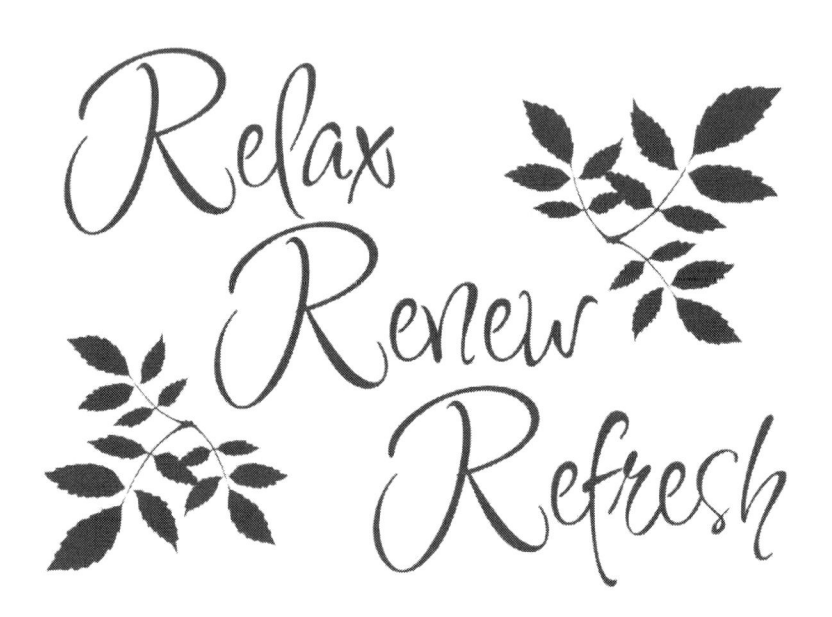

Relax
Renew
Refresh

Day 6: Write Your Vision

Write down your short-term (three to six months) and long-term (one year or longer) fitness goals and create a plan of action needed to reach these goals. Get descriptive and provide measurable means to track your progress.

Day 6 Journal Entry Date:

Short Term Goals:

Long Term Goals:

Day 7: Have a night out on the town

Today you are going to make plans to have a "Girl's Night Out." This is not a suggestion, it is an order. Blow the dust off your heels, call up a few of your friends and plan a great night out. On your night out, do not talk about your beautiful kids, job or wonderful spouse. This is a time for you to disconnect and reconnect with others.

Day 8: Break Free

Today we are going to make plans to adventure somewhere new. I do not know about you, but sometimes I feel stuck in a rut and need to get out of it. Traveling the same route to work every day, doing the same tasks at work and going through the routine of a normal day can get boring.

Do you ever feel this way?

When was the last time you took a different route to work?

What about the last time you went to your favorite restaurant-- did you order the same meal?

Break free and do something unusual today.

Sister to Sister Tip: Getting Out doing New Things and relaxing Will Give You A Brighter Perspective On Life!

Day 9: Ready for Change

Today we are going to reflect on days one through eight. Be honest with yourself about what you have discovered regarding your personality, self-image, childhood experiences, dreams, and goals.

Decide whether you are at a point in your life where you can commit to making a change. Take time; do not rush through this process.

If you cannot take the first step by yourself, find someone you trust to help you move forward. I have learned it is great to have support when we are going through tough moments in life.

Day 9 Journal Entry Date:

Honest Reflection: Write about your discovery

Day 10: New Beginning

Welcome to day 10!

Today is a celebration of a new life! Old behaviors, negative attitudes, and negative thought patterns are being kicked out the door. No longer will you allow other people to define who you are and you are working on changing any negative behaviors you have discovered. You will no longer base your happiness on your clothing size or the numbers on the scale. You are empowered by taking the time to love and care for your body. It is a new day and a newer you. Take what you have learned over these 10 days and continue to work on who you want to become from a mental, emotional, spiritual and physical standpoint.

Continual Quest

It is essential to remember that when it comes to self-discovery, there is no plateau. The search for meaning and purpose is a continuum throughout our lives and if we ever decide to stop searching, our growth will become stagnant.

Changing your health goes deeper than just changing your eating patterns and exercising more.

Therefore, throughout your growth process, continue to set new and challenging fitness and personal goals. smile more often and don't be afraid to look in the mirror at the real you. The stage lights are off and it is safe to remove the mask for good.

The new you is confident, fit, empowered, and ready to take on the world one day at a time.

A Never Ending Covenant

As you continue on this health quest, I want you to make a vow of commitment to yourself.

Making a vow of commitment to yourself will keep you striving every day to live up to the promises you have made to YOURSELF!

CHANGING THE NORM

Why Not Commit to Yourself?

When we get married, we give vows to our future spouse. We speak these vows in front of God, friends, and family and try to uphold every one of them - so why can't we make vows to ourselves and uphold them?

We can and should be encouraged to do so.

Therefore, you can use the vowels I have written to myself, or write your own.

Once you have written your vows, display them in a place where you can see them on a daily basis.

You can place them on your bathroom mirror, your refrigerator or at the office - it's your choice, just make sure this paper is visible and on the days you are not feeling great about yourself, you will have a written reminder of your greatness.

Rehearse your vows in your mind and bind them around your heart by carefully pondering and applying them to your daily life.

Greatness is in you, do you believe it?

Sister to Sister Tip: Committing To Love Yourself Is The Best Decision You Can Make. You're Worth It!

CHANGING THE NORM

Vows of Self-Love

1. I will always love and respect myself.
2. I will laugh at myself when I make mistakes and be kind to forgive myself.
3. I will never settle for less than my worth.
4. I will love myself body and appreciate all it does for me.
5. I will always be honest with myself.
6. I will push myself when I feel like giving up.
7. I will not look at my past and allow it to define my future.
8. I will be my best friend, biggest fan and greatest encourager.
9. I will take time each day to devote to my health, spirit and emotions.
10. I will not be defined by what I do, my body or my bank account

Sister to Sister Tip: Learning To Love Yourself Is A Lifelong Journey. Enjoy The Process!

PART 2
FUEL YOUR SUCCESS

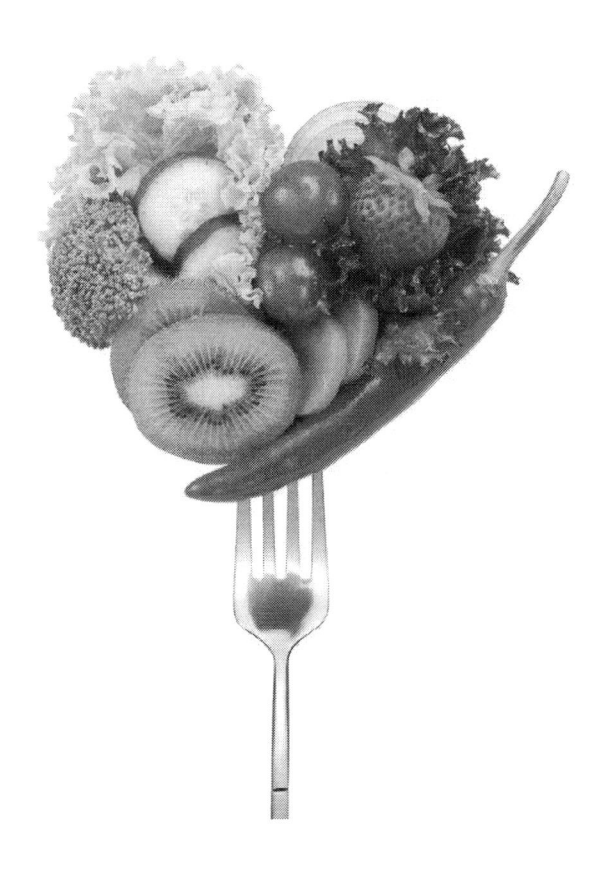

Chapter 9

You Are What You Eat!

You are what you eat!

How many times have you heard this saying?

I would guess too many times to remember. However, my question to you is - have you ever thought about the true meaning of this statement? If you haven't, now is the time to do so.

Is Tradition Killing Us?

For years in the African American community, food has been used as a bridge to connect family and friends.

We eat to celebrate birthdays, marriages, deaths, births, church events and the list goes on.

Celebrating important moments in our lives with food isn't a negative thing. However it's the food choices we make that are placing our community at risk for various chronic health issues.

Hearing me say this may be a little uncomfortable to hear, but as I mentioned in the introduction, I am going to be transparent and encourage you to change the "NORM" of what has always been a part of our culture.

Therefore let's have more sisters' talk about the unhealthy foods in our community!

What About Grandma and Great Grandma?

In past generations, our great, grandparents ate what was provided to them. This often meant eating the leftovers of an animal (Chitterlings, Pigs Feet, etc.) and sometimes limited access to other healthy and nutritious foods.

As years went by, these food traditions were passed down from generation to generation and remain staples in many African American homes and communities.

Therefore, it is essential that we look at our traditions and determine if our traditions are killing us!

CHANGING THE NORM

What's Wrong with Tradition?

I can't count the number of times I've attended a family gathering and have been offered a plate full of traditional staples. These staples smell and look amazing; however, my eating regimen normally doesn't consist of foods rich in gravies, high in sodium, sugar or fried.

I don't eat many of these foods due to my body's reaction after eating them, not because I don't love and appreciate my cultures foods.

By no means am I saying it's wrong to love these foods. However, what I am saying is," It's time to re-evaluate our food choices and their effect on our health."

So where am I going with all of this?

It is my desire to acknowledge the impact tradition on many of the food choices we make for ourselves and our families. As the Matriarch of your family and community, you play a major role in improving the health of your community and family and it starts in YOUR kitchen.

Change Starts in YOUR Kitchen

I believe it is safe to say that the majority of women within the African American community do at least 85 to 90 percent of the meal planning and cooking in their household.

Do you understand what that equates to?

It equates to POWER!

Power to change the "NORM" in your kitchen!

You have the power to turn UNHEALTHY into HEALTHY!

How Do You Use Your KITCHEN POWER?

One way to create POWER in your kitchen is to make your own food instead of feeding your family premade and processed meals (Roman Noodles, Hot Dogs, and canned Meats etc.).

Making your own food gives you the ability to control the ingredients you use and helps limit the amounts of sodium and calories eaten.

Let's use an example!

If you and your family enjoy spaghetti, instead of eating canned spaghetti, you can make your own by using ground turkey, whole-wheat pasta and low sodium spaghetti sauce.

Using lean ground turkey instead of regular hamburger meat can cut down on your consumption of red meat. Using whole-wheat noodles will assist you in feeling fuller which can decrease your desire to consume additional food in one setting. Using Olive Oil and salt-free seasonings can provide your food with flavor without the health risks of using too much bad fat or sodium.

Let's look at another example of kitchen POWER!

You can control the amount of sodium you use in your foods. Numerous African American food staples such as Zatarain's Rice contains high amounts of sodium.

Sodium or salt used in excess in our food has been linked to the increase of hypertension or high blood pressure in African American women.

No one enjoys bland foods, therefore to add flavoring to your food, add olive oil, herbs and spices instead of using table salt. This method can be applied to all of your favorite foods.

Last example!

Do you love fried chicken?

If you do, you don't have to completely get rid of it, instead of deep frying it in unhealthy oils, why not oven fry it in Olive Oil?

Do you see where I am going with all of this!

I'm excited just talking about it.

You can eat healthily and enjoy it. It's all about Kitchen Power! In the recipe chapter of this book I provide you with healthier options for some of your favorite foods!

Slow Down Lady!

I just presented you with a lot of choices didn't I?

I don't want to overwhelm you, but I do want to educate you and show you that you don't have to give up everything you enjoy at the mercy of being healthy.

I understand change is a process, but making small changes such as these on a weekly basis will add up to better health in the long run.

Therefore take one week at a time to add a new healthy habit and before you know it, healthy living will become second nature to you!

To get you started in the right direction and before moving to the next section, take time and read my Top Five Healthy Eating Guidelines.

Top 5 Healthy Eating Guidelines

Follow my top five healthy eating guidelines and you will be well on your way to healthier eating and living!

1) **Prepare foods in advance:** Preparing food in advance will provide you with healthy foods available at all times (work and home). This will help minimize the impulse to stop for fast food or other unhealthy snacks when you're hungry. Portion off healthy snacks and carry with you at all times. Purchase snack sized bags to keep you aware of your portions.

2) **Eat every two to three hours**: Eating small meals more frequently throughout the day will keep your blood sugar levels even and ward off hunger. Eating more frequently will, also help you avoid consuming too many calories at one meal.

3) **Drink water throughout the day**: Over 65 percent of your body is water. Consuming water throughout the day will keep you full and help transport toxins and waste from your body and help curb hunger.

4) **Snack in between meals:** Snacking in between meals will keep the hunger monster away and prevent you from consuming large meals at one sitting.

5) **Limit eating out:** Eating out can be expensive and add inches to your waistline and hips. Therefore, if you decide to eat out, eat out only 1 time per week and go to places that have healthier options on their menu.

To consume fewer calories, request to have salad dressings given on the side and when given large portions, divide portions into two sections. At all times be aware of your portions and don't be afraid to ask for a to-go box for remaining portions.

Following these five tips on a regular basis will assist you in developing healthier habits and keep you more mindful of how much and what you are eating.

Chapter 10

Don't Believe the Hype

Learning how to eat healthy can be a mystery. There are so many products on the grocery market shelves whose packages boast their products to be healthy when in actuality many of these products aren't as healthy as their packaging would like to boast.

Therefore if you're going to get healthy, you have to understand how to determine what is really healthy, from what's not healthy!

Don't let food marketing hype fool you.

Allow me to teach you how to avoid this food label marketing hype!

It's all in the Marketing!

Marketing companies often create extraordinary visuals to grab consumer's eyes. This method of marketing can create a great opportunity to entice consumers with beautiful packaging and fancy words without really telling what's completely in a food product.

What's even more alarming, a lot of marketing of unhealthy products are made to minority children.

Therefore if you have children, more than likely you have fallen for this marketing hype at least once in your life.

Let me show you how this all works.

Grocery Shoppers Lane

Take a moment and walk with me down grocery shopper's lane.

One day you find yourself wandering down the grocery aisle and you pass by a bottle of fruit juice.

Based on its enticing words like 100 percent Daily Serving of Vitamin C and that big buzz word, ANTIOXIDANTS, you grab the bottle of fruit juice and place it in your cart without reading the nutrition or ingredient label.

CHANGING THE NORM

The pretty picture of fresh fruit splashed across the bottle gave you a sense of fruit heaven and if you had a glass available, you would have poured yourself a serving or two.

You finally make it home and want a glass of your fruit juice, but before pouring a glass you turn the bottle over to read the nutrition label and you find your fruit juice really isn't all fruit juice.

At the top of the bottle, you see a sign that says it contains 10 percent fruit juice.

Oh no!

You mean this beautiful bottle really doesn't contain all the fruit it claimed by its array of pretty fruit on the front of the bottle?

You got it, and you have just bought into marketing hype.

Don't feel bad, you are not alone.

Many people buy food items based on what they see the front package instead of turning over the products and reading the nutrition and ingredient labels.

No worries, long gone are the days when you pick up a food product and think it's healthy based on the appearance of the package.

It's time to learn how to read nutrition and ingredient labels.

Let's Make a Deal!

Here's the deal!

You have to agree with me on something! Are you ready? I want you to agree that you will NOT put a food item into your grocery cart without first reading the ingredient and nutrition food label!

Is that a deal? Did you say deal?

Great!

Yes, it will make grocery shopping a few minutes longer; however, you're worth it!

Let's LEARN!

Read All Labels

What are nutrition facts and ingredient labels?

Nutrition facts and ingredient labels are labels located on food products that list nutrients by their daily percentages and ingredients by their weight.

Making the decision not to read these labels and strictly depend on advertisement alone can be misleading. Learning how to read these labels will empower you to know what you are really consuming. Let's learn how to read ingredient and nutrition labels.

Explore the Labels

As you learn to eat healthier, a new guideline for grocery shopping involves not placing any food items into your cart without first reading the nutrition facts and ingredient list label. If it's an unpackaged product (such as fresh fruit or vegetables), it's OK to place these items into your cart. Sticking to this guideline will keep you be more aware of the food choices you are making and help you get accustomed to reading food labels. Yes, this may be more time-consuming, but your health is worth it.

Where do you begin?

First, locate the nutrition facts label on the product. The majority of products list this information either on the back or side of the food item. The nutrition facts label informs you of the amount of a certain nutrient you will consume from a particular product (protein, saturated fat, sodium). Once you have located this label, proceed to follow these steps.

Locate the serving size and the number of servings in the package. Serving sizes are standard to compare similar foods. They are listed in units, such as cups or pieces, followed by the metric unit, e.g. the number of grams. Pay close attention to serving sizes. The more servings in the package equal more calories consumed.

Locate the amount of calories per serving. If you find a package that says 250 calories, but you fail to see that the entire package has two servings and eat the entire package, you are getting 250 more calories for a total of 500 calories.

Look at calories and percentages of fat, carbohydrates, protein, sodium and cholesterol. The nutrition facts label will list these items in grams per serving. Follow your guidelines when it comes to fat. The majority of your calories should come from unsaturated fat. Limit products that are high in saturated and trans fats. In addition to these bad sources of fat, stay away from foods that are high in sodium. Foods with more than 20 percent of your daily value of sodium should be avoided.

Look at the percentages of vitamins and minerals. Underneath the list of macronutrients, you will find a list of vitamins and minerals with their percentages. These percentages are based on the amounts food in the food item.

Once you have read the nutrition facts label, you will look for the ingredients list label. Legally, every food product is required to list all ingredients that were used to make the particular product. Food products normally list ingredients by weight, therefore by reading the ingredient list you are more aware of what is truly in a product.

If you were reading an ingredient list, you would focus on the first five ingredients. Since ingredients are listed by weight, the products that are listed first on the list are the bulk of the product. If the first ingredient is sugar, most of that product is sugar. Even though the nutrition label may state that there are only seven grams of sugar in this product, pay attention to the ingredient list. I stress again, if sugar is the first ingredient on the list, the majority of the product is sugar.

When reading ingredient lists, a rule of thumb to remember is if you can't pronounce the word, more than likely it is a chemical or preservative and you don't want that in your body.

Try to find products that have shorter ingredient lists and are as natural as possible. By doing this, you lessen the chance of putting excessive amounts of unhealthy products in your body.

An example of a food ingredient list may look like this:

Ingredients: sugar, water, salt, high fructose corn syrup, partially hydrogenated vegetable oil

Information that must be listed on all food product packaging includes:

- ✓ Product information
- ✓ A list of ingredients
- ✓ Name of food
- ✓ Net weight
- ✓ Nutritional content
- ✓ The name and address of the manufacturer

Chapter 11

Friend vs. Foe

You have learned a lot of information in the previous chapters, therefore, let's take a moment to exhale.

Whew.

Alright, is your mind clear?

If it is, let's continue to move forward.

We need to move forward and talk about something that keeps many African American women from reaching their fitness and weight loss goals.

We need to address is your relationship with food.

Many African American women find themselves in a vicious cycle of a love-hate relationship with food.

Some are dieters who go through a constant battle with weight gain and weight loss, only to find themselves lost in a sea of disappointment and pounds heavier.

At the other end of the spectrum, there are those who desire to enjoy food but are too consumed with the fear of gaining weight. As a result, they either purge (bulimia) or deny themselves food (anorexia).

Although bulimia and anorexia are often associated with other races and ethnicities, research shows an increase in eating disorders amongst African American women and African American teens.

Therefore, if you or someone you know is currently dealing with an eating disorder, please do not feel alone. There are other African American Women who suffer with eating disorders and you can find help for this condition.

The following organizations can help you with the tools to overcome this often debilitating and often stigmatized condition.

National Eating Disorder Association (NEDA)

www.nationaleatingdisorders.org

Eating Disorder Hope

www.eatingdisordershope.com

CHANGING THE NORM

Do you fit into either one of these categories?

If you do, it is important to realize that you have the power to start a healthy relationship with food.

Eating should be an enjoyable process, but for this to happen, it is essential that you get to the root cause of why you and food have the relationship that you have.

Maybe you're an emotional eater and learned these eating habits during your childhood. If you're an emotional eater, you will be challenged with learning new ways to cope with your emotions. This may require counseling to assist you in your discovery.

It is important you learn how to use food to fuel our bodies and not to suppress or address emotions. It may be scary to address the issues you suppressed, but doing so will free you from this pattern of behavior and allow you to become one step closer to living a healthy life.

If you are struggling with food, find someone you can confide in and let them be your support system, this support system may include a licensed psychologist who specializes in eating disorders or it could mean a spiritual counselor who can pray with you and guide you to a more spiritual path to discover the reasons why behind your eating patterns.

After being honest with yourself and sharing this information with someone you trust, you may discover the root cause(s) of why you feel the way you do about food.

Sister to Sister Tip: Understanding Your Relationship With Food Will Help You Make Better Food Choices and Identify Food Triggers

Chapter 12

No More Dieting

Regardless the number of commercials you see promising drastic weight loss overnight, diets and diet pills don't provide you with PERMANENT weight loss.

They are a Band-Aid to a long-term problem!

Yes, a Band-Aid and we are saying

good- bye to this "NORM"!

Therefore, in this chapter you will learn the importance of healthy nutrients, identify their function in your body, discover how to eat healthy well-balanced meals and learn how to make healthy behavior changes that can ultimately lead to permanent weight loss.

Why Most Diets Don't Work

Before we learn how to eat healthy, let's explore the top reasons why diets don't work!

Most diets are restrictive: Restricting certain foods groups from your nutritional plan may cause your body to miss out on essential nutrients. Restricting these essential nutrients may cause certain health problems if absent from your diet for too long.

Most diets severely decrease your caloric intake: The body requires a certain amount of calories to perform the basic functions of life such as breathing and digestion. Consuming low amounts of calories can cause your body to use other sources such as your muscle tissue (protein) for energy. Very low calories diets can ultimately disrupt your metabolism and in the long run, may actually make it harder to burn calories and lose weight.

Diets are unrealistic and difficult to follow: Choosing to stay on a diet for an extended amount of time is unrealistic. With low amounts of food intake and restriction, diets are often short lived and lead to additional weight gain. You can't eat grapefruit for the rest of your life.

Diets have regimented meal plans: Regimented diets often require the dieter to either buy expensive diet shakes, meals, or stock up their fridge with very specific regimented foods. This can be costly and boring to the palate, leaving you wanting foods higher in calories and flavor.

Most diets make you dependent on prepackaged meals: Numerous diet plans require you to purchase their foods products as a tool for weight loss. In the long run, this can hinder you from learning how to cook, prepare and determine proper portion sizes of food. No one can remain on diet products forever, and eventually you have to learn how to eat in the real world.

The next time you see a commercial promising you permanent weight loss with the popping of a few pills and only three minutes of exercise a day, turn the channel and don't believe the HYPE!

Let's move on and have nutrition talk!

Sister to Sister Tip: Diets Are Short-Term Fixes To Long-Term Problems

Chapter 13

Protein the Building Blocks

Protein the Building Blocks

Although there are many nutrients important to your health, three nutrients make up the majority of your nutritional requirements. These nutrients are termed "macro-nutrients" and includes protein, carbohydrates, and fats.

Macro-fit

When consumed in balance, macro-nutrients provide the body with proper nutrition for the growth and repair of your body's tissues and can provide you with sufficient nutrients to help fight off certain illnesses.

Out of the three macronutrients, there's great confusion about the role of protein. Therefore, protein will be the first macro-nutrient we discuss. We will discuss protein requirements, sources and the role protein plays in getting fit.

Protein: The Building Blocks

Protein is one of the most popular macros. Everywhere you turn - whether it's in a women's health or fitness magazine or on a commercial - there's constant talk about the latest and greatest sources of protein.

Before I go any further, I promise I'm not going to give you a chemistry lesson on protein, but I will provide you with basic information.

What's the truth about protein?

Protein is the major functional and structural component of all cells in the body. Everything from skin, hair, nails, enzymes and collagen are formed from individual proteins (amino acids).

If not consumed in adequate amounts, there's risk of hair loss, skin problems, stunted muscle growth and many other health-related issues. Therefore to keep is basic; protein is needed in your everyday life for all of your body's functions, including repairing muscles from resistance training and exercise.

CHANGING THE NORM

Let's move forward by allowing me to clarify some of the confusion on protein, below you will find frequently asked questions accompanied with the answers regarding the role of protein in regards to getting fit.

FAQS Regarding Protein

Q. HOW MUCH PROTEIN DO I REALLY NEED?

A. The amount of protein you consume is based on your current lifestyle, age, sex, and fitness goals. If you are a sedentary person (inactive), your requirements are lower versus the requirements of someone more active who resistance trains.

For those women who aren't as active, it is recommended that you consume at least 0.8 grams of protein per kilogram of body weight per day.

For more active women who resistance train and desire to build lean muscle, your intake will be higher. For optimal recovery, consume at least 1.0 gram of protein per kilogram of body weight.

No worries, I will show you how to determine your body weight in kilograms.

Use the following equation to determine these samples of protein intake. (See below)

Protein Equation:
Plug in your body weight

Example: If you weigh 150 pounds and are inactive (sedentary)

1. Divide your body weight by 2.2.

    This will convert pounds into kilograms (150/2.2) = 68 kilograms

2. Multiply 68 kilograms by 0.8

    (68x 0.8)= 54

3. Consume approximately 54 grams of protein per day

Q. HOW CAN I ADD PROTEIN TO MY DIET?

A. Protein can be found in foods such as beans, nuts, eggs, dairy products, fish, bison, lean beef, and seafood. When choosing meat, look for sources that are low in amounts of saturated fat*. If you are often on-the-go, purchasing a protein powder and a shaker bottle can provide you with a quick and easy way to get optimal consumption of protein. Just add one to two scoops of protein based on the grams per serving, add water, shake and go.

Saturated fat content is generally located on the nutrition label of the package. Look for items that have less than 5 percent of the Daily Value (DV) from saturated fat

Q. I'M VEGAN, HOW CAN I GET PROTEIN?

A. You can get your required protein intake by consuming a variety of grains, beans, legumes, soy, tofu, veggie burgers and nuts. The key to your protein consumption is to consume a variety and combination of these food items.

Q. WHAT ARE ESSENTIAL AND NON-ESSENTIAL AMINO ACIDS?

A. There are 20 amino acids needed for proper functioning of the human body. Of these 20 amino acids, 8 are considered essential. Essential means the body does not produce them; therefore they must be consumed in the diet. The other 12 amino acids are non-essential, which means the body naturally produces them. To find out more information on amino acids visit www.webmd.com.

Q. WHAT IS THE BEST FORM OF PROTEIN POWDER?

A. There are many forms of protein powder, but whey protein has one of the highest biological values (BV). Biological value is defined by the amount of protein that is readily available and used by the body. You can find whey protein in many nutrition and health food stores.

To find a whey protein that works for you, experiment with different brands and flavors. Whey protein is a by-product of milk, therefore if you are lactose intolerant; this may not work well with your digestive system. If this is the case, you may want to use soy protein or find a whey product that has reduced lactose or is lactose free.

Q. WHAT IS A COMPLETE PROTEIN?

A. A complete protein is a protein that contains all 20 amino acids needed for the body to function properly. Most animal products are sources of complete proteins, whereas plant proteins do not contain all essential amino acids.

Q. SHOULD I CONSUME PROTEIN AFTER A WORKOUT?

A. Yes. It is important to replenish the body with protein (amino acids) after a training session. Consuming protein within 30 to 45 minutes after a workout is important for muscle tissue repair and recovery. After your workout, consume at least 25 grams of protein with a fast absorbing carbohydrate (sports drink such as Gatorade™, PowerAde™, or fruit). Some studies believe combining protein and a fast absorbing carbohydrate will transport amino acids into the cells at a faster rate. Faster delivery equals faster recovery.

Q. WHAT ARE QUICK AND CONVENIENT WAYS TO CONSUME PROTEIN?

A. Purchasing RTD's (Ready-To-Drink) (which are pre-packaged protein drinks) is a quick and convenient way to meet your protein needs. RTD's come in various brands and flavors. These drinks may be pricey, but are convenient.

Before purchasing, read ingredient and nutrition labels. Reading these labels will help you determine the amount of calories, carbohydrates, protein and fat per serving in each drink. Some of these drinks are high in calories and sugar so read ALL labels.

Another convenient way to consume protein is to purchase a tub of protein powder along with a shaker bottle. You can purchase snacks bags and measure out the required amount per serving and place in your gym or lunch bag. The only thing required to make a protein shake is water and a shaker bottle. Shake, enjoy and go!

Q. IF I CONSUME MORE PROTEIN, WILL I GET INTO SHAPE FASTER?

A. No. Consuming more protein will not get you in better shape at a faster rate. A combination of resistance training, regular cardiovascular activities and healthy eating are required to reach optimal health and fitness levels. Protein is used to help build and repair damaged tissue, but consumption alone will not get you to your desired fitness level faster.

Protein Sources

Chicken	Edamame (soybeans)
Beans	Egg whites
Tofu	Lean Beef (93%)
Nuts and Seeds	Fish (Salmon, Halibut, Tilapia)
Peanut Butter	Ground Turkey
Buffalo	Cottage Cheese
Venison	Almond Butter

Fish

Tilapia	**Whiting**
4 oz. 100 kcal	4 oz. 77 kcal
2.5g fat	2g fat
20g protein	18g protein
Cod	**Flounder**
4 oz. 80 kcal	4oz 120 kcal
3g fat	6g fat
14g protein	17g protein
Wild Alaskan Salmon	**Canned Tuna**
4 oz. 80 kcal	(In water or olive oil)
1.5g fat	5 oz. 50 kcal
16g protein	1g fat
	11g protein

CHANGING THE NORM

Deli Meats (low sodium)

Turkey Breasts	Roast Beef
6 slices 50 kcal	6 slices 50 kcal
1g fat	2g fat
8g protein	10g protein
Ham	**Chicken Breasts**
6 slices 50 kcal	6 slices 50 kcal
1g fat	1g fat
9g protein	9g protein

Chicken

Chicken Breast	Ground Chicken
4 oz. 120 kcal	4 oz. 180 kcal
22g fat	11g fat
19g protein	19g protein

Beef

Lean ground beef 93%
4 oz. 180 kcal
8g fat
24g protein

Turkey

Turkey breast cutlets	Turkey Bacon (low sodium)
4 oz. 120 kcal	1 slice 35 kcal
0.5g fat	3g fat
28g protein	2g protein
Ground Turkey	**Turkey Sausage**
4 oz. 140 kcal	2 oz. 100 kcal
3.5g fat	5g fat
27g protein	8g protein

Chapter 14

Fat Attack

The second macro-nutrient we will discuss is dietary fat or fat.

Over the years, dietary fat has earned a negative reputation due to increased health issues related to the consumption of saturated and trans fats in most American's diets, especially diets of the African American community.

Saturated and trans fats (bad fats) have been linked to alarming rates of obesity, heart disease and other health related issues, but all fats are not created equal and dietary fat isn't solely to be blamed for increasing rates of obesity in the African American female population.

Some Fat is Good for You!

Believe it or not, there are good sources of dietary fat and it is important to understand that almost all foods have some form of fat, but the fats you want as a part of your regular nutritional plan are unsaturated fats, which include monounsaturated and polyunsaturated fat. Sounds like a mouthful doesn't it? Allow me to explain.

Monounsaturated and polyunsaturated fats when eaten in moderation are known to provide the body with many health benefits such as lowering your bad cholesterol (LDL), increasing your good cholesterol (HDL), and fighting inflammation. They get their names based on their chemical structure.

The Department of Health and Human Services (H.H.S.) recommends no more than 20 to 35 percent of your diet come from fat.

This means the majority of your dietary fat should come from unsaturated fat, which includes monounsaturated and polyunsaturated fat (examples fish, Olive Oil, Nuts, and Seeds)

The Good, Bad and the Ugly

Understanding the difference between healthy and unhealthy fats is important if you desire to make healthier food choices for you and your family.

Therefore, let's discuss the four major categories of dietary fat which include unsaturated fat, trans fat, monounsaturated fats, and polyunsaturated fats.

CHANGING THE NORM

Unsaturated fats (which include monounsaturated and polyunsaturated fats) are considered healthy sources of fat which have been shown to help lower your risk of heart disease by lowering your bad cholesterol (low-density lipoprotein) (LDL) and increasing your good cholesterol high-density lipoproteins (HDL). Unsaturated fats are found in foods such as nuts, seeds, olive oil and peanut butter.

One polyunsaturated fat known to be beneficial to your health is Omega-3 Fatty Acids. Studies have shown that Omegas 3's appear to decrease your risk of Coronary Artery Disease (C.A.D.) and may protect against irregular heartbeats and help lower blood pressure levels.

Now that we have discussed the categories of healthy fat (good fat) let's discuss the two categories of unhealthy fats (bad fats). The two categories include saturated fats and trans fats. These fats have been linked to causing heart disease, diabetes, and other major health concerns. Food sources that contain saturated and trans fats include baked goods, cakes, pies, red meat cheese and diary. It is recommended that you eat these foods sparingly due to the health concerns linked to their consumption.

Can you avoid dietary fat? No and neither should you try. Instead of completely removing dietary fat from your meals, focus on consuming healthy sources of fat found in products such as nuts, freshwater fish, peanut butter (in moderation), nuts, seeds, olive oil and avocados.

It is also important to understand that although good sources of fat are needed in your nutritional plan when compared to other macronutrients, fat contains more calories per gram

(nine calories per gram).

Therefore, consume in moderation.

FAQS Regarding Fat

Below you will find answers to questions most frequently asked about dietary fat.

Q. WHAT IS SATURATED FAT?

A. Saturated fat is an unhealthy fat found in many foods such as meat, eggs, cheese, fried foods, crackers, cookies, desserts, whole milk, palm oil, and coconut oil. Animal fats are the primary source of saturated fat and should be consumed in moderation.

The U.S.D.A. recommends that less than 10 percent of our total daily calories come from saturated fat. Consuming saturated fat on a regular basis can lead to coronary heart disease and other heart related ailments, therefore saturated fat should be consumed in small amounts.

Q. WHAT ARE TRANS FATS?

A. Tran's fats are unhealthy fats used to preserve the shelf life of many products. trans fats can be found in fried foods, baked goods, chips, cookies and crackers. One common trans-fat is partially hydrogenated oils which are used to keep the crunch in snacks like chips and crackers.

It is recommended that no more than 1 percent of your daily calories come from trans fats. To avoid consuming these fats, read ingredient labels and be aware that some products may list a product as "Trans Fat Free" if a single serving contains less than 0.5 grams. Always read the fine print.

Q. HOW DO I DETERMINE HOW MUCH FAT TO CONSUME?

A. 1. Determine your total calorie intake for the day.

2. Multiply that number by .20 (lower intake of fat) or by .35 (higher intake of fat)

Example: (To figure out the amount of fat you would consume on a daily caloric diet of 2,000 calories: Multiply 2,000 by 0.20 or 0.35 and then divide that number by 9, **(9 equals the number of calories per**

gram of fat.) Based on a 2,000 calorie-a-day diet, this amounts to between 44 to 78 grams.

Fat consumed based on 20%

2000 X .20 = 400

400/9 = 44 grams

Fat consumed based on 35%

2000 X .35 = 700

700/9 = 78 grams

Q. WHAT ARE MONO AND POLYUNSATURATED FATS?

A. Mono and polyunsaturated fats are healthy fats that yield many health benefits when consumed. Foods such as olive oil, fish, seeds, peanut butter and nuts are great sources of healthy fats.

One particularly good fat is Omega-3 fatty acids. Studies have shown that Omega-3 fatty acids have the ability to protect the heart's vessels, prevent inflammation and some forms of Omega-3 are needed for brain, heart and eye health. The majority of your dietary fat should come from sources of mono or polyunsaturated fats.

Q. HOW MUCH DIETARY FAT DO I NEED?

A. It is recommended that no more than 20 to 35% of your total daily calories should come from fat and from mono and polyunsaturated sources.

Guidelines for Fat Consumption:

Saturated Fat: less than 10%

Mono and Polyunsaturated: at least 20%

Trans Fat: no more than one percent

Samples of healthy daily allowances of fat consumption:

1,800 calories a day:

- 40 to 70 grams of total fat
- 14 grams or less of saturated fat
- 2 grams or less of Trans fat

2,200 calories a day:

- 49 to 86 grams of total fat
- 17 grams or less of saturated fat
- 3 grams or less of Trans fat

2,500 calories a day:

- 56 to 97 grams of total fat
- 20 grams or less of saturated fat
- 3 grams or less of Trans fat

Q. HOW CAN I CUT BACK ON EATING BAD FATS?

A. There are many ways to cut back on eating bad or unhealthy fats, which include:

- ✓ Remove skin from chicken, turkey and other poultry before cooking. Skin contains fat.
- ✓ When reheating soups or stews, skim the solid fats from the top before serving.
- ✓ Drink low-fat (1 percent or fat-free (skim) milk rather than whole or 2 percent milk, or almond milk.
- ✓ Purchase low-fat or non-fat versions of your favorite cheese and other milk or dairy products.
- ✓ To satisfy your sweet tooth, reach for a low-fat or fat-free version of your favorite ice cream or frozen dessert. These versions usually contain less saturated fat, but be aware of sugar content in these food

items. The removal of fat sometimes leads to adding additional sugar for taste.

- ✓ Use low fat margarine spreads instead of butter. Most margarine spreads contain less saturated fat than butter. Look for a spread that is low in saturated fat and does not contain trans fats.
- ✓ Choose baked goods, bread and desserts that are low in saturated fat. You can find the fat content on the Nutrition Facts label.
- ✓ Pay attention at snack time. Some convenience snacks (such as sandwich crackers) contain saturated fat. Choose instead to have non-fat or low-fat yogurt, a piece of fruit or lightly salted nuts.
- ✓ Choose leaner cuts of meat that do not have a marbled appearance (where the fat appears embedded in the meat). Choose leaner cuts (including top round and sirloin) and trim all visible fat from meats before eating.
- ✓ Read all food labels and be conscious of what you are eating.

HEALTHY FAT

Polyunsaturated Fats

- Vegetable Oils (Safflower, Corn, and Canola)
- Cold Water Fish (salmon, mackerel)
- Flaxseeds
- Flax Oil

Monounsaturated Fats

- Avocadoes
- Fish (Omega-3 fatty acids)
- Sunflower seeds
- Peanuts
- Olive Oil
- Peanut Butter
- Almonds
- Walnuts

UNHEALTHY FAT

Saturated Fats

- Animal products such as meat, poultry, seafood, dairy products, lard, butter, coconut, palm, and other tropical oils.

Trans Fats

- Partially hydrogenated vegetable oils, commercially-baked goods such as crackers, cookies and cakes, fried foods such as donuts, French fries, shortening and margarine.

Sister to Sister Tip: Not All Fats Are Created. Good Fats Are Essential To Your Health. Eat in Moderation!

Chapter 15

Carbs: The Energy Makers

Carbohydrates are the "rock star" of the bunch! Why?

I will explain why!

Why Rock Star Status?

Carbohydrates, just like fat, have earned a negative reputation over the years due to increased health-related issues such as type 2 diabetes and obesity.

It has been proven that African American's consume excessive amounts of sugar found in processed foods such as cakes, donuts, sugary drinks, white bread and white pasta - which are all devoid of many healthy nutrients.

Consuming these foods is just like opening a bag of sugar and drinking it.

That's a powerful visualization isn't it?

Although the food products just mentioned consist mainly of unhealthy sugars, all sugars aren't bad for your health!

That's right, all sugars are not created equal, and there are healthy forms of sugars.

Therefore let's learn the truth about carbohydrates and healthy forms of sugar!

What Are Carbohydrates?

Carbohydrates are the body's main fuel source that provides energy for basic bodily functions such as breathing, body movements, digestion and normal heart functioning.

When compared to fat and protein, carbohydrates are broken down at a quicker rate and are more readily available for your body to use as energy when compared to any other macro-nutrient.

For many reasons, this is beneficial, but over the years there has been a great amount of dispute regarding whether or not a person should consume carbohydrates or stay away from them.

The Carbohydrate Fad

In the early 2000's, this dispute became profitable for many companies that focused on low-carb diet plans that encouraged low-to-no consumption of carbohydrates but allowed high consumption of unhealthy fats found in meat.

This short-lived diet craze created the buzz that carbohydrates were the enemy within the food industry, but this picture wasn't painted as clear as it should have been.

Why Do You Need carbs?

Have ever been on an extremely low carbohydrate diet?

If you have, you may have experienced low energy levels and restricted mental focus. If this occurred, it was a result of low glucose or blood sugar levels known as hypoglycemia.

As stated earlier, carbohydrates are an important source of fuel for the bodies basic functioning and without the proper amount of carbohydrates from the right sources, the body doesn't function at its best levels.

Why So Much Drama?

Right about now you might be a little confused about carbohydrates because you have always heard carbohydrates are the enemy.

Let me re-emphasize that carbohydrates aren't the enemy and there's no need for you to deal with the carbohydrate drama anymore.

First things first - let's identify the different types of carbohydrates.

There are two primary types of carbohydrates: they are complex carbohydrates (three or more sugar molecules) and simple sugars (one or two sugar molecules).

These two categories of carbohydrates are categorized by the number of sugar molecules they are made of and each type of carbohydrate metabolizes (breaks down) differently in the body based on their chemical structure.

What are complex carbohydrates?

Complex carbohydrates are made up of three or more sugar molecules. This molecular structure results in a slower absorption rate into our blood stream as compared to simple sugars. This slow absorption rate provides the body with sustained amounts of energy and you are less likely to experience the blood sugar spikes compared to consuming simple sugars.

Therefore, it is recommended that the majority of your carbohydrates come from complex carbohydrate sources such as whole-grain bread sweet potatoes, quinoa, brown rice, steel cut oatmeal, and vegetables.

We have learned about complex carbohydrates, now let's learn about simple sugars.

What are simple sugars?

Simple sugars are made up of one or two sugar molecules. Their molecular structure results in faster sugar absorption into our bodies and high spikes in blood glucose or blood sugar levels.

Consumption of simple sugars provides quick, but inadequate, amounts of sustained energy. These sugars are found in processed foods such as baked goods, milk products, honey, corn syrup, molasses, brown sugar and maple syrup.

Consuming high amounts of simple sugars has been linked to diabetes, weight gain and other health-related issues including inflammation. Therefore, these sugars should be consumed in moderation.

The Great Crash

Allow me to show you how eating simple sugars can affect your health!

Let's travel down memory lane for a moment.

Have you ever had one of those mornings where you didn't have time to do anything, including eating a healthy breakfast?

You stormed into work one minute before start time and didn't recognize your hunger signals until you reached your desk and started working.

After working for a few minutes, you listen to your hunger signals and take a quick stroll into the office kitchen where you find donuts and a cup of coffee. You grab a donut, cup of coffee, and indulge in both. All of a sudden, you get this burst of energy and feel like you can attack all of your work in no time.

Before long, you feel like taking a nap and your desk seems like a good place to get some shut-eye.

Can you guess what happened?

You have just experienced a sugar crash!

Bob, tell her what she has won!

Behind door number one, there is a big headache followed by the desire to take a nap and eat more sugar or caffeine to get more energy.

Behind door number two, is a case of Type 2 diabetes from the continual blood sugar spikes.

Finally, behind door number three are 15 to 20 extra pounds that you will eventually see in the mirror and on the scale.

Yikes! I know that wasn't what you expected was it? Remember at the beginning of the book I told you that I was going to be transparent and honest with you? We're sisters, so I'm going to as the young ones say" Keep it real! "

In keeping it real, I want you to be fully aware that eating excessive amounts of simple sugars are detrimental to your health and waistline.

Therefore, it is essential to monitor the amounts and types of carbohydrates you consume on a daily basis, especially if you have diabetes.

How Do You Eliminate Eating Bad Sugars?

First, you can limit the amount of simple carbohydrates (unhealthy) or sugars in your diet by ensuring you always have healthy snacks and meals prepared for the workday.

Having healthy snacks like fresh fruit, nuts, veggies and lean protein will assist you in making better food choices within your work day.

Second is to be mindful of the types of drinks you consume this includes fruit juice. Although fruit juice can be a healthier option compared to drinking soda, fruit juices contain high amounts of sugar.

Therefore, if you choose have 100 percent fruit juice instead of a soda, make sure you read the label and if possible stick with juices like Juicy Juice that typically on have 10-12 grams of sugar per serving based on flavor.

CHANGING THE NORM

Third, consume white pasta's, noodles and white breads in moderation. These foods are processed or stripped and breakdown quickly into your body and can spike your blood sugar levels.

By using these three steps you can remain mindful and more aware of your sugar intake.

Be Aware of Condiments

Also don't forget to make sure you read the food labels on Spaghetti Sauce, Ketchup and BBQ Sauces, these condiments have a lot of hidden sugars!

Rank Your Carbohydrates

Now that you have learned the basic essentials about carbohydrates, let's learn one way to ensure you are eating the right types of carbohydrates.

This can be accomplished by learning how to use the glycemic index.

What is the Glycemic Index?

The "Glycemic Index" is a numerical ranking system which assigns a numeric value to foods based on their immediate rise or effect on blood sugar levels.

Foods with a high ranking of 70 and above enter into the blood streams quickly, whereas foods with a ranking of 55 and lower enter into the blood stream at a lower and steady rate.

Foods with a high ranking (70 or above) should be eaten sparingly and the majority of your carbohydrates should be chosen from the low ranking category in order to maintain healthy blood sugar levels, weight and to lessen your chance of getting Type 2 diabetes.

In order to use the glycemic index to make healthier food choices, familiarize yourself with the numbers of the foods you currently enjoy eating.

If you discover that the majority of your foods come from the higher ranked category, start to discover new foods that appeal to your liking from the lower ranked carbohydrate list.

Getting used to new tastes may be a challenge, but in the long run will be beneficial to your health.

Below you will discover a glycemic index for over 100 foods.*

Food	Glycemic Index (glucose = 100)	Serving Size (grams)	Glycemic Load per Serving
BAKERY PRODUCTS AND BREADS			
Banana cake, made with sugar	47	60	14
Banana cake, made without sugar	55	60	12
Sponge cake, plain	46	63	17
Vanilla cake made from packet mix with vanilla frosting (Betty Crocker)	42	111	24
Apple, made with sugar	44	60	13
Apple, made without sugar	48	60	9
Waffles, Aunt Jemima (Quaker Oats)	76	35	10
Bagel, white, frozen	72	70	25
Baguette, white, plain	95	30	15
Coarse barley bread, 75-80% kernels, average	34	30	7
Hamburger bun	61	30	9
Kaiser roll	73	30	12
Pumpernickel bread	56	30	7
50% cracked wheat kernel bread	58	30	12
White wheat flour bread	71	30	10
Wonder™ bread, average	73	30	10
Whole wheat bread, average	71	30	9
100% Whole Grain™ bread (Natural Ovens)	51	30	7
Pita bread, white	68	30	10
Corn tortilla	52	50	12
Wheat tortilla	30	50	8

BEVERAGES

Coca Cola®, average	63	250 mL	16
Fanta®, orange soft drink	68	250 mL	23
Lucozade®, original (sparkling glucose drink)	95±10	250 mL	40
Apple juice, unsweetened, average	44	250 mL	30
Cranberry juice cocktail (Ocean Spray®)	68	250 mL	24
Gatorade	78	250 mL	12
Orange juice, unsweetened	50	250 mL	12
Tomato juice, canned	38	250 mL	4

BREAKFAST CEREALS AND RELATED PRODUCTS

All-Bran™, average	55	30	12
Coco Pops™, average	77	30	20
Cornflakes™, average	93	30	23
Cream of Wheat™ (Nabisco)	66	250	17
Cream of Wheat™, Instant (Nabisco)	74	250	22
Grapenuts™, average	75	30	16
Muesli, average	66	30	16
Oatmeal, average	55	250	13
Instant oatmeal, average	83	250	30
Puffed wheat, average	80	30	17
Raisin Bran™ (Kellogg's)	61	30	12
Special K™ (Kellogg's)	69	30	14

CHANGING THE NORM

GRAINS			
Pearled barley, average	28	150	12
Sweet corn on the cob, average	60	150	20
Couscous, average	65	150	9
Quinoa	53	150	13
White rice, average	89	150	43
Quick cooking white basmati	67	150	28
Brown rice, average	50	150	16
Converted, white rice (Uncle Ben's®)	38	150	14
Whole wheat kernels, average	30	50	11
Bulgur, average	48	150	12

COOKIES AND CRACKERS			
Graham crackers	74	25	14
Vanilla wafers	77	25	14
Shortbread	64	25	10
Rice cakes, average	82	25	17
Rye crisps, average	64	25	11
Soda crackers	74	25	12

DAIRY PRODUCTS AND ALTERNATIVES			
Ice cream, regular	57	50	6
Ice cream, premium	38	50	3
Milk, full fat	41	250mL	5
Milk, skim	32	250 mL	4

Reduced-fat yogurt with fruit, average	33	200	11
FRUITS			
Apple, average	39	120	6
Banana, ripe	62	120	16
Dates, dried	42	60	18
Grapefruit	25	120	3
Grapes, average	59	120	11
Orange, average	40	120	4
Peach, average	42	120	5
Peach, canned in light syrup	40	120	5
Pear, average	38	120	4
Pear, canned in pear juice	43	120	5
Prunes, pitted	29	60	10
Raisins	64	60	28
Watermelon	72	120	4
BEANS AND NUTS			
Baked beans, average	40	150	6
Blackeye peas, average	33	150	10
Black beans	30	150	7
Chickpeas, average	10	150	3
Chickpeas, canned in brine	38	150	9
Navy beans, average	31	150	9
Kidney beans, average	29	150	7

Food	Glycemic Index (glucose = 100)	Serving Size (grams)	Glycemic Load per Serving
Lentils, average	29	150	5
Soy beans, average	15	150	1
Cashews, salted	27	50	3
Peanuts, average	7	50	0
PASTA and NOODLES			
Fettuccini, average	32	180	15
Macaroni, average	47	180	23
Macaroni and Cheese (Kraft)	64	180	32
Spaghetti, white, boiled, average	46	180	22
Spaghetti, white, boiled 20 min, average	58	180	26
Spaghetti, whole meal, boiled, average	42	180	17

Food	Glycemic Index (glucose = 100)	Serving Size (grams)	Glycemic Load per Serving
SNACK FOODS			
Corn chips, plain, salted, average	42	50	11
Fruit Roll-Ups®	99	30	24
M & M's®, peanut	33	30	6
Microwave popcorn, plain, average	55	20	6
Potato chips, average	51	50	12
Pretzels, oven-baked	83	30	16
Snickers Bar®	51	60	18
VEGETABLES			
Green peas, average	51	80	4

CHANGING THE NORM

Carrots, average	35	80	2
Parsnips	52	80	4
Baked russet potato, average	111	150	33
Boiled white potato, average	82	150	21
Instant mashed potato, average	87	150	17
Sweet potato, average	70	150	22
Yam, average	54	150	20
MISCELLANEOUS			
Hummus (chickpea salad dip)	6	30	0
Chicken nuggets, frozen, reheated in microwave oven 5 min	46	100	7
Pizza, plain baked dough, served with parmesan cheese and tomato sauce	80	100	22
Pizza, Super Supreme (Pizza Hut)	36	100	9
Honey, average	61	25	12

* "International tables of glycemic index and glycemic load values: 2008" by Fiona S. Atkinson, Kaye Foster-Powell, and Jennie C. Brand-Miller in the December 2008 issue of Diabetes Care, Vol. 31, number 12, pages 2281-2283.

CHANGING THE NORM

Below are answers to some of the most frequently asked questions regarding carbohydrates.

FAQs Regarding Carbohydrates

Q. WHAT WILL HAPPEN IF I GO TOO LONG WITHOUT CARBOHYDRATES?

A. Going too long without a sufficient amount of carbohydrates will cause the body to find other sources of energy to function. This energy may come from protein (muscles) or fat stores. Going long periods of time without a sufficient amount of carbohydrates can cause fatigue and dizziness. The brain and central nervous system need carbohydrates (glucose) in order to function properly, therefore consume carbohydrates in moderation and in the form of complex carbohydrates (whole grains, beans, brown rice and legumes).

Q. SHOULD I CONSUME CARBOHYDRATES BEFORE I WORK OUT?

A. Yes. Carbohydrates are the body's main source of energy and the amount you consume before a workout is based on your fitness goal. If your goal is to build lean muscle, you'll need to consume at least 45 to 50 grams of carbohydrates along with 10to 15 grams of protein. If your goal is weight loss, consume at least 25 grams of carbohydrates and 15 grams of protein.

If you're going to consume your carbohydrates in a liquid form, consume it at least 45 minutes prior to your workout. If your source is whole food, allow 90 minutes to two hours for food to digest before training. If you exercise for more than an hour, you may need to refuel with a sports energy drink such as Gatorade™ or PowerAde™ in order to maintain energy levels. On non-work out days, carbohydrate consumption should be lower. On these days, the body doesn't require as much energy to fuel your body.

Q. WILL CARBOHYDRATES MAKE ME FAT?

A. No, not if consumed in moderation and in the form of complex carbohydrates, along with regular physical activity and resistance training. People don't become overweight by just consuming carbohydrates. Weight gain is a combined result of consuming too many calories and limited physical activity.

Q. IS IT ALRIGHT TO CONSUME SUGAR-FREE PRODUCTS?

A. Many sugar-free products contain high amounts of synthetic or artificial flavoring and studies have shown some products may cause diarrhea and gastric problems such as bloating and gas. Instead of consuming artificial sweeteners, opt for natural sweeteners that have zero calories. Stevia™ and Truvia™ are a few.

Q. IF I DON'T WANT TO USE REFINED SUGAR, WHAT IS A GOOD ALTERNATIVE TO SWEETEN FOOD?

A. There are many natural products on the market such as agave nectar, Stevia™ and Truvia™ that add flavoring and don't cause high sugar spikes. Most of these products are at your local grocery or health food store. You may use these products to bake or sweeten your favorite drinks.

Q. WHAT IS THE PERCENTAGE OF CARBOHYDRATES SHOULD I CONSUME DAILY?

A. The amount of carbohydrates you consume on a daily basis is based on your daily physical activity, fitness goals and current weight. If you are an athlete, your intake of carbohydrates may be between 50 to 60 percent or higher based on the intensity and duration of your activity. For less active individuals, at least 40 percent of your diet should come from complex carbohydrate sources.

Q. HOW DO I CALCULATE THE GRAMS OF CARBOHYDRATES I NEED TO CONSUME ON A DAILY BASIS?

A. The first step in calculating your required grams is to determine your fitness goals. Do you want to lose weight or do you want to focus more on athletic events and gaining lean muscle? If you want to lose weight, take 40 percent of your daily calories to determine carbohydrates in grams. If you want to build lean muscle tissue or you're an athlete, take at least 55 percent of your daily calories.

Example: You want to lose weight and you consume 1,600 calories a day

1. Take 1,600 X .40 = 640
2. Take 640/4 (4 = the amount of calories in 1 gram of carbohydrates) = 160
3. Your total daily consumption of carbohydrates equals 160 grams

Example: You want to gain lean muscle or you're athletic and you consume 2,200 calories a day

1. Take 2,200 x. 55 = 1211.
2. Take 1,221 / 4 (4 = the amount of calories in 1 gram of carbohydrates) = 302.5
3. Your total daily consumption of carbohydrates equals 302.5

CHANGING THE NORM

Daily Caloric Tracking Sheet

One way to become aware of how much you're eating and determine the amounts from each food group is to journal or track your meals. This sheet will also allow you to monitor your moods before and after your meals, this may help identify food triggers. Make copies and create a journal.

Sun:	Mon:	Tue:	Wed:	Thu:	Fri:	Sat:

Weight: **Date:**

Weekly Eating Goal(s)

Place	Time of Day	Food/ Beverage	Calories	Mood Before	Mood After

Daily Calorie Intake:

What were you feeling today? (Happy, sad, excited, bored, lonely, angry, depressed, jealous, determined, persistent etc.)

Water consumption:

Daily Overview (triggers you discovered, patterns in eating, types of foods most craved, etc.):

Do You Have A Healthy Relationship With Food?

Take time to answer each question honestly. The answers to these questions are for your eyes only and may reveal important information to you regarding your eating habits and patterns.

Date:

1. Do you skip breakfast on a regular basis?
2. Do you eat even when you are not hungry?
3. Do you eat when you are happy, sad, bored, and alone or excited?
4. Do you listen to your body's hunger signals or do you ignore them?
5. Do you feel bad about eating in front of others?
6. Do you enjoy fresh fruits, whole grains and veggies regularly?
7. Are you frequently on a diet?
8. Do you consume too many empty calories (alcohol), soda or energy drinks?
9. Do you eat every 2-3 hours?
10. Do you deny yourself food when you are hungry?
11. Do you eat while working?

Research shows stress is a possible trigger point for emotional eating. Therefore if you find you're a stress eater, it will be essential to find new and healthier ways to deal with your stress such as going for a walk, or dance class.

We all have stressors, we just have to discover healthy ways to cope with them!

Chapter 16

As you continue your fitness and health journey, pack these tools in your purse!

Tools for Success

- ✓ **Never skip breakfast:** Skipping breakfast will cause you to become hungry throughout the day and consume extra calories. Therefore start your day off right by having a healthy breakfast.

- ✓ **Always keep healthy snacks available:** Keeping healthy snacks available will keep you from eating office junk food or visiting a snack machine whenever you are hungry. Use snack bags to portion off snacks like fresh cut fruit, vegetables and nuts.

- ✓ **Increase your fiber intake.** Fiber keeps you full and helps regulate healthy bowel movements. Fiber is the indigestible part of food that helps remove waste from the digestive track.

- ✓ **Do not eat when bored or stressed:** Emotional eating can add pounds to your frame. If you are going through a tough time, take a minute before you eat and ask yourself are you hungry or are you eating to sooth a particular emotion. If you're not hungry, go for a brisk walk or find a good book to read.

- ✓ **Eat small, frequent meals throughout the day every 2-3 hours:** Eating frequently throughout the day will prevent hunger and drops in your blood sugar levels.

- ✓ **Limit your amount of alcohol.** Alcohol is full of empty calories and can increase caloric intake. Drink sparingly and in moderation.

- ✓ **Eat complete meals:** Eating a complete meal involves including a source of protein, fat and a complex carbohydrate (whole grains). Eating complete meals will keep you full longer and provide your body essential nutrients.

- ✓ **If you have a family, make a group decision to make healthier food choices:** A rule of thumb: if you shouldn't eat unhealthy food, neither should your family. Making a family decision will make the transition easier and beneficial to the entire family.

- ✓ **Be aware of food portions:** Eating large portions of food can cause weight gain. Therefore, purchase a weight scale and weigh your food until you train your eye to determine true size proportions. Eating with smaller plates can help give you a visual aid.

- ✓ **If you fall off the health wagon, start over fresh the next day:** If you get off track with your healthy eating, don't throw in the towel. Guilt will not help get you back on track. Address your barriers and move forward.

- ✓ **Limit your intake of processed and canned foods:** Processed and canned foods contain high amounts of sodium and chemicals which, if consumed in large amounts, can lead to water retention (edema) and high blood pressure (hypertension). Limit these products and purchase fresh or frozen.

- ✓ **When grocery shopping, shop the perimeter of the store:** By shopping on the perimeter of the grocery store you will find fresh fruits, vegetables, and other healthy products. Shopping in the middle aisles is where the majority of processed and canned foods are located.

- ✓ **Always read nutrition labels:** Read all nutrition facts and ingredient list labels. Don't be fooled by pretty packaging and creative wording.

- ✓ **Consider food as fuel for the body. Look at food as fuel and this will help you make better food choices:** Without proper fuel (food) the body doesn't function the way it was designed and you gain excessive amounts of weight.

- ✓ **Prepare meals in advance:** Preparing meals in advance will help you avoid making impulsive food decisions. Try to avoid leaving your house without healthy meals or snacks on a daily basis.

- ✓ **Take time and chew your food slowly:** Chewing your food slowly will allow you to enjoy the taste of your food and give you a sense of fullness. Don't eat while working, step away from your work and enjoy your food.

- ✓ **Avoid foods high in saturated and trans fat:** Consuming foods high in saturated and trans fat can lead to high cholesterol, heart disease, obesity and many other health risks. Eat these foods sparingly.

- ✓ **Use condiments sparingly:** Ketchup and creamy salad dressings can be high in sugar and calories and offer little-to-no nutritional value. Get creative and make your own seasonings by using herbs, olive oil and sea salt.

CHANGING THE NORM

- ✓ **Start each meal with small amounts of food on your plate:** Start off by eating small amounts of food. Eat what is on your plate and then take a few minutes to decide if you are still hungry. If the answer is yes, then go back for another small portion of food.

- ✓ **Choose lean sources of protein:** Lean sources of meat have less fat and are healthier. Therefore, choose sources at least 93 % lean.

- ✓ **Choose complex carbohydrates:** Choosing complex carbohydrates such as whole grains, brown rice, quinoa, and steel cuts oats over simple sugars (cakes, donuts, and crackers) can help maintain your blood sugar levels and ward off the hunger monster.

- ✓ **Buy frozen or fresh fruits and vegetables:** Buying foods that are fresh or frozen or in their most natural state are healthier than boxed or processed foods. Eat boxed and processed food sparingly.

- ✓ **Reduce sodium intake:** Consuming high amounts of sodium can cause health issues such as hypertension. Therefore, instead of using salt, season food with spices and herbs. If you choose to use salt, sea salt is a healthier alternative.

- ✓ **Drink sufficient amounts of water:** More than 60 percent of the body is made of water. Water is used for weight loss, to carry nutrients to cells, cushion joints and to regulate body temperature and blood pressure. Therefore, consume at least 2.2 liters (nine cups per day). If you exercise, drink water before, during and after your workouts. Being dehydrated (lack of water intake) can cause fatigue and affect your optimal exercise performance

Chapter 17

It's a Family Affair

Creating healthy meals for yourself can be challenging, however creating healthy meals for you and your family can become even more challenging especially in today's fast-paced busy world.

NO Fast Food Please!

As a busy mom, drive-thru may seem more convenient, but do not be fooled by amazing marketing from fast food companies who promote healthy options. Fast food isn't healthy for you or your family.

It's All About Marketing

As I mentioned in an earlier chapter, research shows many well-known food chains advertise unhealthy foods to kids, and especially to minority children.

Recently there have been health policies and regulations that attempt to limit the degree of advertisement geared toward children.

However, as a mother you need to be aware that if a particular food isn't healthy for your body, it isn't healthy for your child's body either.

I understand fast food is easy and if you're a single mom, your boat runs over. However, imagine how stressful it would be having an obese child.

Childhood Obesity in on the Rise!

Whether you're single or raising your family with a partner, I need to emphasize childhood obesity within the African American community is on the rise.

According to the National Health and Nutrition Examination Survey, 35.9 percent of African American children are obese.

That's a very alarming statistic and what's even more alarming is that children who are obese are more than likely to become adults who are obese and have obesity-related health conditions.

In addition to health conditions associated with obesity, obese children are known to suffer from emotional stress due to being bullied by other children.

CHANGING THE NORM

I know you love your children and the mere thought of this may break your heart. However, if we are going to change the "NORM", we must see our truths and work on changing them.

Resistance Will Be Felt!

I will be 100 percent honest and tell you that changing the eating habits of your family won't be easy!

The hardest barriers to overcome is having children eat healthier when they have become accustomed to eating unhealthy flavorful foods.

Although you may get resistance from your children, understand change is a process for them as well. Therefore it will require you to be patient and understanding, yet firm with your food decisions.

Besides, you and your family deserve to eat meals that nourish your body and health. At times it may seem impossible to change both you're eating habits and your family's, however, keep in mind that even if your family isn't ready to change their eating habits, stay committed to the promises you've made to yourself.

As your family makes positive changes don't forget to congratulate them on any step they take towards healthier living. By doing this, you are showing your family that you value their efforts even if they aren't as committed as you are.

Remember, you have the POWER to start changing the "NORM" in YOUR household!

Healthy on a Budget

Although the economy is slowly improving, families and singles continue making budgets cuts. Unfortunately, some of these budget cuts are being made to grocery bills.

Do you find yourself in this situation?

If you find yourself with a limited grocery budget, it's normal for you to believe healthy eating is too expensive. Although there is some truth to this statement, it is possible to find ways to purchase healthy food for yourself and your family while still keeping your budget.

CHANGING THE NORM

Allow me to share a few tips with you!

1. **Buy in Bulk**: Buy in bulk by purchasing a Sam's or Costco card. If you can't buy a Costco card on your own, split the price with another person. Buying food items in bulk saves you money per item. Be aware that when buying in bulk, avoid buying perishable items unless they can be placed in the freezer to eat at a later time. Buying too much perishable food will go fast and, in the process, cause you to lose money.

2. **Clip Coupons**: Clipping coupons is tedious work, but it will save you money. Therefore create a surplus of coupons and use them as often as possible.

3. **Search for Grocery Depots and Outlets**: Grocery depots and outlets provide selected brand items and some name brand items at a lower the normal prices. When purchasing these items, be sure to check expiration dates on all items. Food items are typically discounted lower when they are close to their expiration date. If you find fruits on sale, check them for bruises. Only buy fruit that looks healthy on the outside.

4. **Price Compare:** Make a list of all the items you need to prepare your meals and determine where you can find the items you need for the cheapest price. You may discover your meat products are less expensive at one store versus another store. Use this method for your produce, veggies, and fruits. Some stores will price compare on certain items.

5. **Create a Grocery List**: Creating a grocery list is a necessity when grocery shopping on a budget. Therefore, before heading out to the grocery store, look throughout your cabinets and freezer to take inventory of what you have. From this point, you can make a menu based on what you need. Having a grocery list will save time and money by preventing you from buying unnecessary food items. It's okay to buy a few wants, but when on a budget focus on what you need! When creating a grocery list, it should be made with specific meals in mind. Making meals at home is far less expensive than investing in pre-made and prepackaged food items. Create a menu plan for the week and stick to it. Meal and menu planning resources can be found online at http://www.whatscooking.fns.usda.gov/. The library is also great resource for recipes, meal ideas, and menu planning. You can check books out without the thought of fees.

6. **Buy local**: Locate a farmer's market within a close proximity of your residence. Most farmers' markets are held on weekends and are cheaper than buying from a large grocer. Your fruits and veggies may also be fresher due to limited transport. Buy veggies and other produce on sale and freeze the portions you and your family don't consume right away. Freezing your food right away has been shown to lock in nutrients. If you don't have transportation, get with your local church and request a bi-weekly bus trip to be organized to take you and others to the farmers markets. Many farmers take EBT cards.

Healthy On a Budget CAN Be Done!

Although it may seem overwhelming to provide a healthy lifestyle for you and your family, don't allow the THOUGHT that healthy costs too much defer you from applying these tips.

Remember your health EMPOWERS every aspect of your life. You and your family are worth finding ways to get healthier!

Additional Sites to Locate Healthy Meal Ideas

Choose My Plate: www.choosemyplate.gov

Eating Well: http://www.eatingwell.com/

Cooking Light: http://www.cookinglight.com/

All Recipes: http://www.cookinglight.com/

Whole Foods Market: http://www.wholefoodsmarket.com

Chapter 18

Feed the Machine

It's Not a Diet, It's a Lifestyle

This chapter provides you with easy to prepare, palate pleasing recipes for breakfast, lunch, dinner and snacks. The nutritional content and calories counts for each meal are listed on each recipe card. In order to give you a generalized idea of what to eat within a day, a sample meal plan for 1,600, 1,800 and 2,000 calorie meal plans is provided. Do not forget to eat every 2-3 hours and track your meals to determine your daily caloric intake.

Eat, enjoy and thrive!

Breakfast

Breakfast is the most important meal of the day and shouldn't be skipped. Eating a balanced amount of calories during this time of the day will fuel your body for the remainder of the day and leave you less hungry. Studies have shown people who eat breakfast on a consistent basis are more likely to manage their weight. The meals below provide you with variety and flavor.

Below are your options for breakfast.

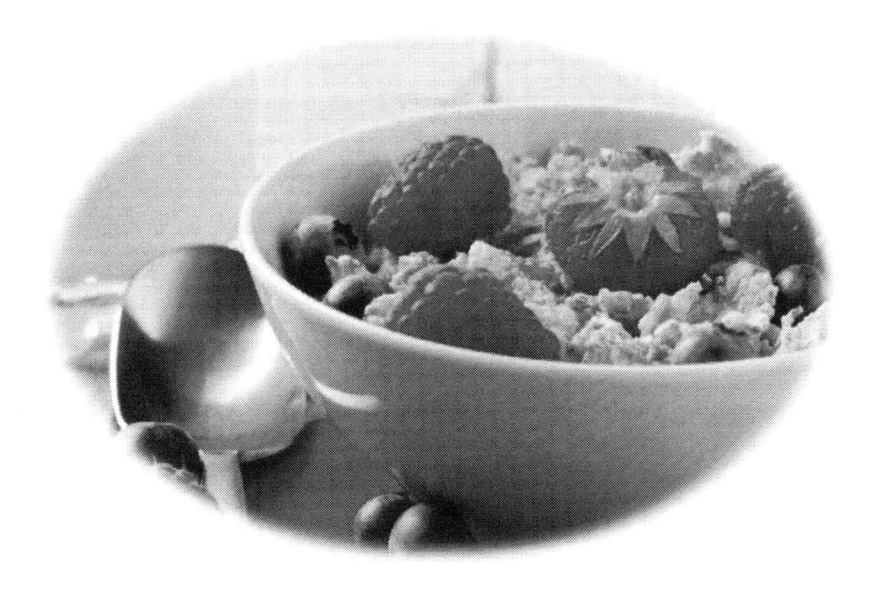

CHANGING THE NORM

CINNAMON NUT OATMEAL

Ingredients:
½ cup Steel Cut Oatmeal
½ oz. Slivered Almonds
Cinnamon (use to your liking. Cinnamon has many health benefits minus the calories)
Agave Nectar (few drops)

Preparation:
1. Boil 1 cup of water and place oats into water.
2. Cook for 3-5 minutes.
3. In a bowl, add slivered almonds, a few drops of Agave Nectar and cinnamon and mix together.
4. Once oatmeal is cooked, place mix on top.

Total calories 232, protein 8 g, carbohydrates 29.8 g, fat 1.5 g

To add more protein, add two egg whites to meal for an additional 34 calories and 7 g of protein.

PUMPKIN SPICE FRENCH TOAST

Ingredients:
1 or 2 pieces of Ezekiel Bread
1 whole egg
2 egg whites
Pumpkin Spice
Nutmeg
Few drops of Agave Nectar
Pam nonstick spray

Preparation:
1. Crack one whole egg and two egg whites into a bowl, add cinnamon and nutmeg, then mix.
2. Place bread into egg mix. Allow each side to absorb mix for about 1 minute.
3. Use a medium sized skillet, cover bottom of pan with Pam. Add bread to skillet.
4. Cook on each side until brown. Once done, add a few drops of Agave Nectar on each side in the pan. Allow bread to caramelize before taking out of skillet.

Total calories 220, protein 12 g, carbohydrates 30, fat 5 g

To add more protein to this meal, add 3 slices of low-sodium turkey bacon 35 calories per slice equals 105 kcal.

BREAKFAST BURRITOS

Ingredients:

2 whole eggs
1 egg white
½ bell pepper
½ tomato
½ onion
1 whole wheat tortilla
Pam nonstick spray
1 slice non- fat cheese
2 Tbsp. salsa
Salt and pepper

Preparation:
1. Chop bell pepper, tomato, onion, and place in a bowl.
2. Crack whole eggs and egg white into bowl with veggies; add salt and pepper, mix.
3. In a medium size skillet, cover bottom of skillet with Pam non-stick spray and add egg mix.
4. Scramble until eggs are to your liking.
5. Take tortilla and add fat-free cheese, place egg mix on top then wrap. Place salsa on top (optional).

Total Calories 300, protein 14 g, carbohydrates 19 g, fat 12g

Add 2 slices of low sodium bacon that adds another 70 calories. You may also add ½ glass of all natural 100 percent fruit juice.

BREAKFAST BAGEL

Ingredients:
1 whole wheat bagel
2 egg whites
3 tomato slices
1/2 slice fat-free cheese ½
Tbsp. light mayonnaise
Pam nonstick spray

Preparation:
1. Spray skillet with Pam non-stick spray. Crack egg and cook until done
2. Slice tomato into 1 inch slices.
3. Cut bagel in half and place in toaster until browned. Remove bagel from toaster and spread light mayonnaise onto both pieces of bread. Add cheese and tomatoes on one-half.
4. Once egg is done add egg to bagel.

Total Calories 340, protein 15g, carbohydrates 35 g, fat 6.5 g

Lunch or Dinner Choices

The following meals can be eaten for either lunch or dinner - you make the choice. Just like breakfast, don't skip lunch.

Lunch

Lunch is a time to refuel your body for the remainder of the work day, which will help stave off the hunger monster and your cravings for unhealthy snacks.

If you are like most people who enjoy eating out during the workday, plan ahead and make wise food choices. Call the restaurant ahead of time in order to determine if they offer a healthy options menu. By doing this, you can plan what you are going to eat before your arrival to the restaurant. If portion sizes at the restaurant are large, don't be afraid to ask for a to-go-box and split half of your meal for later.

NUTRITION JEWEL

Fuel your midday with a healthy lunch and avoid the mid-day hunger monster

Dinner

Dinner is the last full meal of the day and shouldn't consist of more than 350 calories. By this time of the day, if you have eaten every 2-3 hours, the hunger monster shouldn't be too hard to handle. If you have missed eating your required calories during the day, be aware of the amount of calories you consume before bedtime. Eating a large meal will pack the pounds on. If you are hungry before bed, have a light snack and drink a glass of caffeine free tea or water to give you a sense of being full. When choosing meals for dinner time, it is recommended to choose meals that are lower in carbohydrates. As the body slows down its activity level towards the latter part of the day, we don't need as many carbohydrates. All calories that are not used as energy are converted and stored as fat. Therefore, be aware of your caloric intake before bed.

Enjoy these flavorful and palate pleasing recipes and don't be afraid to add extra vegetables for more nutrients and fiber.

NUTRITION JEWEL

When you Eat great, You feel great & look great!

TUNA QUESADILLAS

Ingredients:
1 -5 oz. can tuna (in water)
Whole wheat tortilla
½ cup tomatoes
½ scallions
2 Tbsp. salsa
½ Tbsp. of mayonnaise
1 slice fat-free cheese

Preparation:
1. Drain tuna, mix mayonnaise with tuna.
2. Chop tomatoes and scallions.
3. Spray skillet with non-stick Pam spray. Place one tortilla in skillet then place tuna mix in middle of tortilla.
4. Add cheese on top of tuna mix. Add second tortilla on top. Brown one side then flip to other side. Cut quesadilla into four triangles. Add salsa on top.
5. Add a side salad with fat free dressing and plenty of veggies to complete meal.

Total Calories 345, protein 21g, carbohydrates 32 g, fat 12 g

In order to cut back on calories, only consume half of quesadilla and prepare 2 servings of vegetables which is 1 cup of vegetables of your liking. You may also prepare a salad to add with half serving

TUNA MELT

Ingredients:
1- 5 oz. can tuna (in water)
½ Tbsp. mayonnaise
2 slices whole wheat bread
2 slices tomatoes

Preparation:
1. Drain tuna, add mayonnaise, mix.
2. Lightly spread olive oil spread on both sides of bread. Place bread in heated skillet. Place tuna mix in middle of bread and place tomatoes on top of mix. Place second piece of bread on top.
3. Cook until brown on both sides. Brown both sides to your liking. Cut in half and serve.

Total calories 406, protein 33g, carbohydrates 40 g, fat 10 g

To cut back on carbohydrates and calories, use thinly sliced bread or a pita pocket.

CHANGING THE NORM

TURKEY BURRITOS

Ingredients:
4 oz. ground turkey
1 whole wheat tortilla
½ chopped tomato
½ onion
1 slice fat-free cheese
½ Tbsp. olive oil
1 Tbsp. sour cream
2 Tbsp. salsa

Preparation:
1. Add ½ Tbsp. of olive oil to a heated skillet. Season turkey meat with selected seasoning, and then add meat to skillet. Once meat begins to cook, add onions. Brown meat until fully cooked.
2. Slightly brush olive oil on front and back of tortilla. Place tortilla in microwave for 20 seconds. Do over cook or tortilla will become too hard.
3. Take tortilla and place fat free cheese in middle, add turkey mix, then wrap.
4. Place chopped tomatoes, fat-free sour cream and salsa on top of wrap.

Total calories 440 calories, protein 38g, carbohydrates 35 g, 9.5 g fat

For less calories, cut burrito in half and save remaining half for later.

TURKEY EXTRAVAGANZA

Ingredients:
4 oz. Turkey Sausage
2/3 cup whole wheat Penne pasta
½ green pepper
½ red pepper
½ red onion
2 Tbsp. fat-free Italian Dressing
1 Tbsp. olive oil

Preparation:
1. Heat water until water comes to boil. Add pasta and cook for 5-7 min. Do not overcook pasta.
2. Cut sausage into 1-inch slices. Chop green peppers, red peppers and onions into 1-inch slices. In a medium size bowl, add all ingredients together.
3. Add one Tbsp. of olive oil to a medium sized pan. Once oil is heated, add sausage, bell peppers and onions to pan. Allow mix to sauté for 7-10 minutes. Do not overcook.
4. Once mix is finished sautéing, add two Tbsp. of fat-free Italian dressing and mix.
5. Drain pasta then add mix on top of pasta.

Total calories 450, protein 24 g, carbohydrates 35 g, fat 10 g

CHANGING THE NORM

SPINACH SUNRISE SALAD

Ingredients:
4 oz. Chicken breast
4 cups baby spinach
½ apple
½ cup mandarin oranges
¼ cup walnuts
1 Tbsp. Raspberry Vinegar Dressing

Preparation:
1. Grill or bake chicken and cut chicken into 1-inch slices, or use 4 oz. precooked chicken strips.
2. Chop apples into square pieces.
3. In a bowl mix, walnuts, oranges, apple pieces and salad dressing.
4. Add mix to baby spinach.

Total calories 350, protein 23g, carbohydrates 40 g, fat 3g

SUNDRIED TOMATO WRAP

Ingredients:
1 sun dried tomato wrap
3 slices deli roast beef
3 slices turkey breast
½ Tbsp. Ranch Dressing
3 tomato slices
1 slice fat-free cheese

Preparation:
1. Place cheese on the bottom of tortilla. Place roast beef and turkey breast on top of cheese.
2. Place in microwave for 20 seconds to heat.
3. Spread dressing on top of meat then add tomatoes.
4. Wrap and cut in half.

Total calories 325, protein 24 g, carbohydrates 35 g, fat 11.5 g

CHANGING THE NORM

Snacks

Eating healthy is about moderation, not deprivation.

Snacks can be from 100-200 calories. Snacking in between meals will keep your blood sugar levels stable and help you avoid overeating. Get creative and enjoy!

DARK CHOCOLATE STRAWBERRIES

Ingredients:

½ cup trimmed strawberries
½ dark chocolate
4-5 toothpicks

Preparation:

1. Melt dark chocolate.
2. Thoroughly rinse strawberries and cut off stems.
3. Insert toothpicks into strawberries.
4. Dip strawberries into dark chocolate.

Approximately 100-150 calories, depending on chocolate.

FLAVORED POPCORN

Ingredients:

1 snack bag natural light popcorn
Choice of seasoning (Parmesan, Cinnamon sugar, Cheyenne Pepper, Hot Sauce)

Preparation:

1. Pop popcorn.
2. Sprinkle seasoning onto popcorn, close bag, then shake.

Approximately 100 calories.

CHANGING THE NORM

BAGEL AND CREAM CHEESE

Ingredients:

½ whole wheat bagel
2 Tbsp. fat-free cream cheese (flavored)
1 serving low fat spread

Preparation:
1. Cut bagel in half; wrap other half for later use.
2. Lightly spread low-fat spread on bagel, then place bagel into toaster.
3. Toast bagel until lightly brown. Remove from toaster and add cream cheese.

Approximately 115 calories.

CHOCOLATE RICE CAKE AND PEANUT BUTTER

Ingredients:

2 rice cakes
1 Tbsp. peanut butter

Preparation:
1. Spread ½ tablespoon of peanut butter on each rice cake.
2. Eat and enjoy.

Approximately 175 calories.

HUMMUS AND WHOLE GRAIN CHIPS

Ingredients:

½ cup whole wheat crackers (lower sodium) 2
Tbsp. hummus (plain or flavored)

Preparation:

1. Spread hummus onto whole grain crackers.
2. Eat and enjoy.
Approximately 150 calories.

CHANGING THE NORM

APPLE AND CHEESE STICK

Ingredients:

1 medium sized apple
2% milk string cheese

Preparation:

1. Thoroughly wash apple. Eat apple with cheese.

Approximately 165 calories.

SWEET POTATO FRIES

Ingredients:

1 medium sized
potato Pam non- stick
spray Pinch of salt

Preparation:

1. Preheat oven to 350 degrees for 5-6 minutes.
2. Thoroughly wash outside of potato.
3. Cut potato into fours.
4. Cut each fourth into 1-inch slices.
5. Sprinkle pinch of salt on potatoes and mix.
6. Spray non-stick pan with Pam spray.
7. Add potatoes to pan.
8. Cook until brown. Rotate potatoes once or twice to brown each side.

Approximately 120 Calories.

CHOCOLATE STRAWBERRY SOY SHAKE

Ingredients:

1 cup chocolate soy milk
½ fresh strawberries 4-5
ice cubes (optional)

Preparation:

1. Trim and thoroughly clean strawberries.
2. Pour cup of soymilk into blender. Add strawberries and ice.
3. Blend. Pour mix into cup.

Approximately 125 calories.

To get more protein in this snack, add one scoop of chocolate or plain whey protein.

PEANUT BUTTER HONEY WRAP

Ingredients:

½ whole wheat tortilla wrap
½ medium banana
1 Tbsp. peanut butter
Few drops of honey

Preparation:

1. Cut whole tortilla wrap in half, and then cut banana in half.
2. Spread peanut butter onto tortilla and then spread honey on top of peanut butter.
3. Place banana in middle of tortilla then wrap.

Approximately 225 calories.

Sample Meal Plans

The following meal plans are samples of **1,600**, **1,800** and **2,000** calories. These meal plans are just an example of how to plan your day based on your daily caloric intake.

As a rule of thumb, consume your first meal within one hour from the time you awake and eat every 2-3 hours thereafter. Eating every 2-3 hours will fuel your body on a consistent basis and relieve hunger and cravings.

Sample Meal Plan for 1,600 Calories

Meal # 1
Breakfast: Breakfast Burrito = 220 calories
½ avocado = 60 calories
4 oz. almond milk = 30 calories

Snack # 1
1 small sized apple = 95 calories
1 2% milk string cheese = 70 calories

Meal # 2
Lunch: Sundried Tomato Wrap = 325 calories
1 small garden salad with 1 tbsp. fat–free dressing = 45 calories

Snack #2
1/3 cup serving of almonds = 160 calories

Meal # 3
Dinner: Spinach Sunrise Salad = 350 calories
1 glass decaffeinated tea = 2 calories

Snack # 3
Chocolate Strawberry Soy Shake = 125 calories
1 120-calorie pistachio snack = 120 calories

Sample Meal Plan for 1,800 Calories

Meal # 1 Breakfast: Breakfast Bagel = 340 calories ½ avocado = 60 calories 4 oz. almond milk = 30 calories **Snack # 1** 1 small sized apple = 95 calories 1 2% milk string cheese = 70 calories
Meal # 2 Lunch: Sundried Tomato Wrap = 325 calories 1 small garden salad with 1 tbsp. fat–free dressing = 45 calories **Snack #2** 1/3 cup serving of almonds = 160 calories 5 celery sticks = 75 calories
Meal # 3 Dinner: Spinach Sunrise Salad = 350 calories 1 glass decaffeinated tea = 2 calories **Snack # 3** Chocolate Strawberry Soy Shake = 125 calories 1 120-calorie pistachio snack = 120 calories

A healthy, well-balanced meal with healthy sources of fat, protein and complex carbohydrates are essential to your weight loss and health.

CHANGING THE NORM

Sample Meal Plan for 2,000 Calories

Meal # 1
Breakfast: Banana Nut Oatmeal =
232 calories
2 egg whites = 35 calories
4 oz. almond milk = 30 calories

Snack # 1
1 small sized apple = 95 calories
1 2% milk string cheese = 70 calories

Meal # 2
Lunch: Sundried Tomato Wrap =
325 calories
1 small garden salad with 1 tbsp. fat–free dressing = 45 calories

Snack #2
1/3 cup serving of almonds =
160 calories
5 celery sticks = 75 calories

Meal # 3
Dinner: Spinach Sunrise Salad =
350 calories
1 glass decaffeinated tea = 2 calories

Snack # 3
Chocolate Strawberry Soy Shake = 125 calories
1 120-calorie pistachio snack =
120 calories

Meal #4
½ Turkey Burrito = 220 calories
1 garden side salad = 45 calories

Healthier Cooking Options for Your Health!

To reach optimal health and maintain a healthy bodyweight, it is essential to be mindful of the ingredients you use when cooking your foods. Therefore below you will discover healthier options to replace unhealthy cooking oils, high-sodium seasonings and sugar.

The options below aren't all inclusive therefore purchasing a healthy recipe book will provide you with more healthy cooking options!

Instead of using these oils to cook your foods:

- ✓ Palm
- ✓ Palm Kernel
- ✓ Coconut

Use these Oils:

Canola Oil

- ✓ **Flavor** – Plain and mild
- ✓ **Uses** – Sautéing, baking, frying, marinating

Olive Oil

- ✓ **Flavor** – Extra virgin olive oil: fruity, tangy, and bold. Light olive oil: mild
- ✓ **Uses** – Grilling, sautéing, roasting, spreads for breads, base for Italian, Greek and Spanish dishes
- ✓ **Quick tip** – Drizzle extra virgin olive oil on top of soups, toasted bread, rice and pasta dishes for a rich flavor.

Peanut Oil

- ✓ **Flavor** – Nutty yet mild
- ✓ **Uses** – Stir-frying, roasting, deep frying, baking

CHANGING THE NORM

Sesame Oil
- ✓ **Flavor** –Light sesame oil: nutty. Dark sesame oil: bold and heavy
- ✓ **Uses** – Stir-frying (light only), Dressings/sauces (dark)

Vegetable Oil
- ✓ **Flavor** – Plain and mild
- ✓ **Uses** – Sautéing, baking, frying, marinating

Instead of using table salt to season your foods try using:
- ✓ Herbs
- ✓ Spices
- ✓ Lemons
- ✓ Limes
- ✓ Seasonings that contain less than 50 mg of sodium per serving

Instead of using refined sugar for your baking and other recipes try:

These are alternatives however contain sugars therefore should be used in moderation. High consumption of sugar can increase your risk for diabetes and weight gain.

- ✓ Agave Nectar
- ✓ Stevia
- ✓ Truvia
- ✓ Unsweetened Apple Sauce (baking)

CHANGING THE NORM

Don't Get Rid of Your Traditional Foods, Just Make Them Healthier!

Below is a list of a few traditional staples of the African American diet. Instead of cooking these staples the traditional way, you will discover a newer way to make the foods that connect you and your family together healthier but still soul fulfilling!

Yummy Collards Greens

INGREDIENTS	COOKING INSTRUCTIONS
• 2 pounds greens (turnips & collards) • 3 cups water • ¼ pound smoked turkey breast, skinless or 4 slices of low-sodium Turkey Bacon • 1 tablespoon hot pepper, freshly chopped • ¼ teaspoon cayenne pepper • 1 teaspoon cloves, ground • 2 cloves garlic, crushed • ½ teaspoon thyme • 1 stalk scallion, chopped • 1 teaspoon ginger, chopped • ¼ cup onion, chopped • Onion powder	1. Separate greens and wash thoroughly. 2. Remove stems. 3. Use your hand to tear or slice leaves of greens into bite-sized pieces. 4. Pour 1 tablespoon of Olive Oil into pot 5. Place all ingredients into pot except greens and bring to a boil 6. Once ingredients have come to a boil add greens 7. Allow greens to cook for 20-30 minutes or until tender as desired. 8. Once done add a 2 teaspoons of vinegar for taste.

Make it a Meal: Go meatless and add a serving a beans and another vegetable with these Yummy Collards Greens.

Cooking Option: If you don't want to boil your greens try sautéing them in Olive Oil!

Health Benefit: This staple is typically made with neck bones, ham or other cured meats that are high in sodium. By using healthier low sodium meats and seasonings, this can become a healthier version of what you're used to.

CHANGING THE NORM

Crispy Oven Fried Chicken

INGREDIENTS	COOKING INSTRUCTIONS
- 1 teaspoon low sodium poultry seasoning - ½ cup or buttermilk or almond milk, or fat-free milk - 1 tablespoons onion powder - 1 tablespoons garlic powder - 2 teaspoons black pepper - 1 teaspoon Chili Pepper - 1 cup cornflakes or whole wheat bread crumbs - 6 pieces skinless chicken, Leg Quarters or Drumsticks - ¼ teaspoon paprika - Nonstick cooking spray (use to coat baking pan)	1. Preheat oven to 350 °F. 2. Remove skin from chicken, then wash chicken and pat dry. 3. Mix seasoning in a bag with crumbs 4. Dip chicken into milk, shake to remove excess liquid, then quickly place chicken in a bag with seasoning and crumbs. 5. Once done mixing, refrigerate for 1 hour 6. After removing from refrigerator coat baking pan with nonstick cooking spray and evenly space chicken in pan. 7. Cover with aluminum foil and bake 40 minutes. Remove foil and continue baking for additional time at least 30 more minutes or until meat is tender and fully cooked. Drumsticks may require less baking time than the breasts. 8. Do not turn chicken over. Allow it to cook all the way through without flipping.

Make it a Meal: Serve up this delicious chicken with a side of fresh sliced tomatoes, cucumbers with a vinaigrette salad dressing with basil sprinkled on top! Can you say delicious!

Health Benefit: Instead of frying chicken in unhealthy fats, oven baking provides flavor minus the unhealthy fat that comes from frying.

CHANGING THE NORM

Happy Baked Macaroni and Cheese

INGREDIENTS	COOKING INSTRUCTIONS
- 2 cups whole wheat of regular macaroni - Nonstick cooking spray - ½ cup onions, chopped - ½ cup evaporated, fat-free milk - 1 medium egg, beaten - ¼ teaspoon black pepper - 10 oz. (1¼ cups) fat-free-sharp cheddar cheese, finely shredded - 1 cup of regular or whole wheat bread crumbs - Sprinkle of Parmesan Cheese	1. Preheat oven to 350 °F. 2. Cook macaroni according to package directions. Add a few drops of Olive Oil to water without adding sodium to water. Once done, drain water and set pasta aside. 3. Lightly coat a saucepan with nonstick cooking spray. 4. Add onions to saucepan and sauté for about 4 minutes 5. In a separate bowl, combine macaroni, onions, and the remaining ingredients and mix thoroughly. 6. Lightly coat a casserole dish with nonstick cooking spray. 7. Transfer mixture into casserole dish. 8. Bake for 25 minutes or until bubbly. Let stand for 10 minutes before serving. 9. Add a sprinkle of parmesan cheese

Health Benefit: Using fat-free cheese and fat-free milk makes this traditional side dish healthy, but still full of flavor!

Make it into a meal: By adding 4-6 oz of a lean meat such as a Turkey Cutlet or skinless chicken breast along with 2 servings of fresh vegetables can make this an enjoyable healthy meal!

Hearty Yams

INGREDIENTS	COOKING INSTRUCTIONS
- 3 medium yams (1½ cups) - ¼ cup brown sugar, packed - 1 teaspoon flour, sifted - ¼ teaspoon salt - ¼ teaspoon ground cinnamon - ¼ teaspoon ground nutmeg - ¼ teaspoon orange peel - 1 teaspoon soft tub margarine - ½ cup orange juice	1. Preheat oven to 350 °F. 2. Peel and then cut yams in half, slice into 1/4-inch thickness 3. Fill a pot of water with 2 cups of water and place yams into pot and boil until tender but firm (about 20-25 minutes). 4. Combine sugar, flour, salt, cinnamon, nutmeg, and grated orange peel into a bowl. 5. Coat a medium-sized casserole dish with nonstick cooking spray. Place half of the sliced yams in the dish. Sprinkle with spiced sugar mixture. 6. Add a second layer of yams, using the rest of the ingredients in the same order as above. Add orange juice. 7. Bake uncovered in oven for 20 minutes.

Health Benefit: Using butter instead of margarine is healthier for your heart! **Make it into a meal:** Go meatless and add a serving of black beans and sautéed spinach as sides. Here's to your health!

CHANGING THE NORM

Menu Planning Sheet

Copy the following sheet and use it to plan your weekly meals. Having a plan of action for your weekly meals will keep you focused on clean eating. Get creative and try new healthy foods.

Day: _____ **Date:** _____

Breakfast:
_____
_____
_____
_____
_____
_____

Lunch:
_____
_____
_____
_____
_____
_____

Dinner:
_____
_____
_____
_____
_____
_____

Snacks:
_____
_____
_____
_____
_____
_____

PART 3
YOUR FITNESS JOURNEY

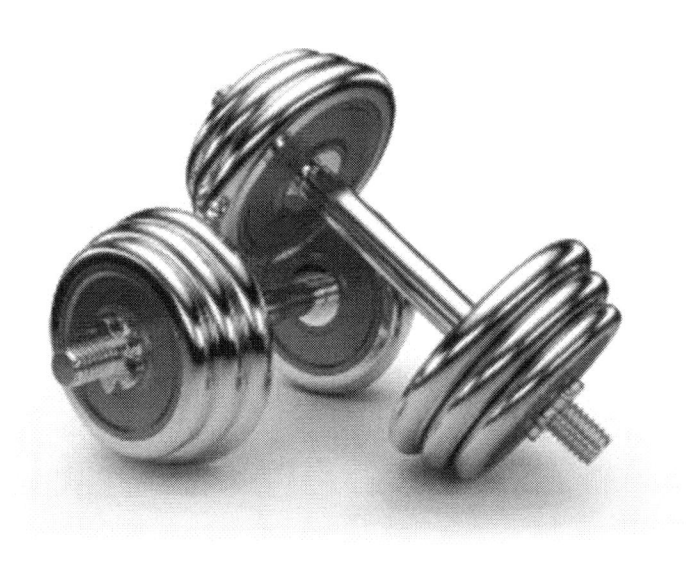

Chapter 19

Let's Address the Barriers!

Beginning a fitness-training or workout program is an exciting life changing adventure, but often, excitement gets replaced with feelings of frustration and confusion.

Feelings of frustration and confusion are often the result of not knowing where or how to start.

Have you ever felt this way?

Where do you go to get what you need?

Although there are possibly thousands of fitness, health, nutrition and wellness books on the market, many of these books do not place an emphasis on the unique needs of the African American.

These books don't address barriers to exercise such as hair maintenance, accessibility to safe parks or gyms and the cost of gym memberships.

Good-bye Statistics!

We can't change all of the barriers that affect the health of African American women on a systemic level (limited access to healthy foods, safer parks, fast food advertisements to inner city kids) but we can change the factors on a individual level (exercise, proper eating and stress management).

Therefore let's discuss the individual factors that are potentially holding you back from getting fit.

Not My Hair!

Up until August of 2011, I was faithful at getting my hair permed every six-weeks.

I'd faithfully go to my stylist and wait hours before she'd call me into her chair, but once in her chair she'd do magic to my hair and I'd always leave her shop with a feeling of hair heaven.

You know what I mean don't you!

That fresh clean smell of newly permed hair that bounced in all the right places!

CHANGING THE NORM

You're smiling! You must know exactly what I mean!

As you know, African American women take pride in our hair and we invest thousands of dollars annually in hair care services (2.7 billion dollars annually) and products.

It's a commendable thing for one to take pride in their hair appearance, however, here's where we have to change the "NORM".

According to a research study published in Archives of Dermatology, *"Hair Care Practices as a Barrier to Physical Activity in African American Women"* more than 40 percent of African-American surveyed admitted to not working out due to their fear of sweating out their expensive hair styles.

First allow me to say that I know exactly how these 40 percent of women feel.

Whenever I permed my hair, I'd always make sure to work out in the mornings before I had my hair appointments with my stylists.

I knew firsthand that by doing my workouts prior to my hair appointment that I was guaranteed to be in hair heaven for at least 48 hours after my hair was permed.

However, two days later, I'd go back to the gym, and good-bye freshly permed hair!

This was a regular occurrence, but I found a solution!

Natural Here I Come!

In August of 2011, I realized that perming my hair was no longer conducive to my fit and active lifestyle.

Therefore within the same month (yes even after spending a lot of money on the first visit to get a perm) I went back to my stylist and asked her to cut all of the perm out of my hair.

I Was Afraid!

I was very afraid to return to my hairs natural state but I knew going natural would be beneficial to my health, my wallet and to my hair.

As I watched my stylists cut my hair, I felt free and nervous all at the same time.

I'd be getting perms since I was a child and hadn't seen my hair any other way.

Therefore questions like, how would I look, what would others think, could I maintain my hair!

I didn't have all the answers to these questions, but nonetheless, I made a decision and I was sticking with it.

Once my stylists cut my hair, I realized my health was more important to me than my permed hair that no longer supported my active lifestyle, therefore, it was time to change my "NORM"!

Stick with Me!

So where am I going with all of this?

Is the moral of my story for you to go all natural?

The answer is NO!

Natural hair isn't for every African American woman, and that is perfectly acceptable.

Therefore, what is the moral of my story? The moral of my story is this! Don't allow the maintenance of your hair to be a barrier or the main reason why you choose not to get fit.

Although it takes more awareness of my hair's condition due to it being natural, I no longer worry about my hair getting sweaty after a workout.

To keep my hair moisturized before and after my workouts, I twist my hair up and spray an all-natural spray on it. I work out just as intensely as I did when I was wearing a perm and don't give my hair a second thought.

After my workouts, I leave my hair pinned up (I don't twist it so tight that it pulls on my edges), spray it again with all natural oils before showering, use a silk wrap before bed and head to sleep.

The next morning I shower and untwist my hair!

Just like that!

Within 20 minutes, I'm ready to head out the door.

Yes, it has become that simple. I reside in Florida and no longer worry about not enjoying the beach due to my hair getting wet and so many other benefits have resulted from being natural!

CHANGING THE NORM

Sure, natural may not be your thing but try the following tips to help you overcome some of your hair concerns.

4 Tips to Break The Hair Barrier!

1) **Wear a Short Style:** If you have long hair try opting for a short style instead. Wearing your hair shorter may require less maintenance and provide you with more time to exercise.

2) **Braids Please**: If done properly, braids can be a great protective style and can help cut down on your hair maintenance time. However, if you opt for this style, remember your hair stills need to stay moisturized to prevent breakage. Also, to keep your hair from thinning avoid wearing braids too tight or constantly in an up do. These styles place tremendous stress on the edges of your hairline.

3) **Go Natural:** Making the decision to go natural after wearing perms for many years can be scary, however, being natural will give you more freedom to stay active without the constant worry of perming your hair. Go to You Tube and watch videos on how to maintain natural hair before doing your big chop to determine if natural is for you.

4) **Up Do:** Getting your hair done in an up do can cut down on maintenance and lessen your chance of having to redo your hair every day for at least two weeks. If you can't afford to have a stylist do your up do, learn how to do an up do on your own!

New Hair can Be Scary!

The thought of changing your hair style my make you uneasy at first, but you are my sister and I have to tell you, choosing a more manageable hairstyle for my active lifestyle has been one of the best decisions I have made and I want to encourage you to do the same.

If you're having doubts about choosing a new style have an open talk with your stylist and also find others who have made the decision to change their hair in order to live a healthier lifestyle!

You can do this, I'm cheering you on!

Chapter 20

I Can't Afford to Get Fit!

Hair maintenance was the first barrier that many African American women face in regards to getting fit, now let's talk about money as a barrier!

Have you ever thought about starting a workout program but once you determined the cost you decided that a gym membership wasn't affordable?

If this is you I have good news for you.

You don't have to go to the gym to get fit. This has been a long standing myth and a detractor for many African American women who aren't in the financial position to join a gym.

Therefore allow me to share a few options that are free or minimal in cost.

The first option is to visit your local library and check out fitness and workout videos. Typically the only thing required is for you to be a resident of your particular county.

Some libraries may charge you if or when you lose your library card but other than that, no fees should be required.

When searching for fitness and workout videos look for videos that capture your interest. If you like to dance, look for the videos that will allow you to dance.

The rule of thumb when choosing any exercise video is that it must be fun and enjoyable. If you enjoy it, you will more than likely desire to do more of that particular activity.

The second option is to find a recreation center in your area or surrounding area. Most recreation centers are free or charge or charge a very low fee to attend fitness classes or to use the facilities weight training room if one is available.

The third option is to start a fitness or walking group at your church. In addition to creating a walking group, you can have a group of your fellow congregants all chip in to have someone come out and teach a fitness class once per week. Most instructors charge no more than $35.00 per hour class.

Therefore, get at least 10 to 12 people and you each chip in to pay for the instructor fee. Paying for an instructor will also increase your level of commitment. It may not be a large sum of money, however, it is a financial commitment on your behalf which shows ownership and interest in your health.

Barriers are Meant to Be Knocked Down!

Using the following tips places you in control of finding a way to exercise by yourself or with a group of others who want to also commit to their health.

I believe we are empowered only when we are given information and apply it to our lives. Yes, we face many barriers in our lives, but barriers are meant to be knocked down!

Sister to Sister Tip: Don't Allow People Or Things In Life To Stop You From Investing In Your Health

Chapter 21

5 Steps to Get CURVElicious

I Don't Want to Look Like a Man!

We have finally arrived at the section where you will find the right exercises to TIGHTEN, TONE, and FIRM your CURVES!

However, before you start picking out exercises in the following chapter, allow me to offer some assurance that you will not look like a man from using resistance training or weight lifting exercises as a part of your fitness training program!

What do I mean?

Allow me to expound for just a second, I promise I won't be too long!

For years women have been led to believe if they lift weights they will become muscular and manly looking. This is far from the truth and I will tell you why!

You WON'T Look Like a MAN

Women naturally have lower levels of a masculine hormone called testosterone. Testosterone is the male hormone that gives men their manly features such as facial hair, deep voices, and dense muscle tissue.

Women possess a small amount of this hormone in their bodies, therefore, most women do not produce large manly muscles from lifting weights.

The chances of getting bulky and manly muscles are slim to none.

However, I do want to educate you and inform you that some women use male hormones and steroids to create larger muscles.

This can often be seen in the body building and fitness world. Once again, I say this with caution, and use the phrase *some* women.

I have reached the highest level of my sport (Fitness Olympia) and have never chosen to use steroids or male hormones. There are many other great female athletes who have excelled in their chosen sport and do not use enhancement drugs.

Now that we have put that old myth to rest allow me to tell you about the many benefits of lifting weights!

Lifting weights can assist you in burning more body fat, building stronger bones, increasing your metabolism and burning calories while at a state of rest!

Yes, you can burn calories at the state of rest! I thought you'd like that one.

With so many benefits of lifting weights, it's hard not to brag on the reasons to try weight lifting.

Over my career, I have been able to use weight training to help sculpt my body and become one of the world's top-ranked athletes.

I'm completely mindful that it may not be your goal to become an athlete, but I do want to encourage you to try lifting weights. By doing so you can transform the shape of your body, create stronger bones and feel empowered by your own strength!

If you feel intimated to start weight training program, hire a personal trainer for a few sessions and allow him or her to teach you the proper way to lift weights.

At first you may feel like a fish out of water, but I am confident that once you see the results and you begin to challenge your mind to push your body harder than you have ever pushed before, you won't be able to put the weights down!

Let's move on and learn five steps to getting fit!

FIVE STEPS TO GETTING FIT

Step 1. Discover Your Body Type

Discovering your body type is an important step in creating an individualized fitness training program to meet your individualized fitness goals. Having an understanding of your body type will help you set realistic goals and expectations and relieve you from trying to make your girlfriend's fitness program work for you.

They are three main body types, which include ectomorph (banana), mesomorph (apple or triangle) and endomorph (bell or pear). It is common for women to be a combination of two body types. Due to your individuality, it is important that you do not compare your body to other women. Your body may be smaller on top and larger on the bottom, or you may be larger on top and smaller on the bottom. Whatever your body type, you have your own unique structural foundation and your training should be tailored accordingly.

CHANGING THE NORM

Below are descriptions of each body type and the recommended resistance and cardiovascular training regimen. Read all descriptions and determine a realistic category for your body type.

ECTOMORPH BODY TYPE

Body Description

Thin body structure, short torso, thin limbs and narrow feet and hands. Has difficulty putting on weight and does not carry a lot of muscles.

Unlike the mesomorph and the endomorph, an ectomorph is a person who has been skinny their entire life. It is not a result of a good diet or strict workout ethics. They are born with a super-fast metabolism which allows their body to break food down at a higher rate. This gives them the "ability" to eat whatever they desire and not gain weight.

Resistance Training

The use of moderately light weights in combination with a repetition range of 12 to 15 can help tone the ectomorph body type. People with this body type may lack strength, therefore if strength is a goal, lifting heavier weight is required (15 pounds or more) to become stronger.

Cardiovascular Activity

Due to the high metabolism of this body type, performing an excessive amount of cardiovascular activity is not advantageous. Performing high amounts of cardio will prevent this body type from developing lean, toned muscles. Therefore performing 30 to 35 minutes of cardiovascular activities will help maintain lean muscle and not promote a stringy appearance and be sufficient to maintain cardiovascular health. Sufficient caloric intake is important to fuel this body type.

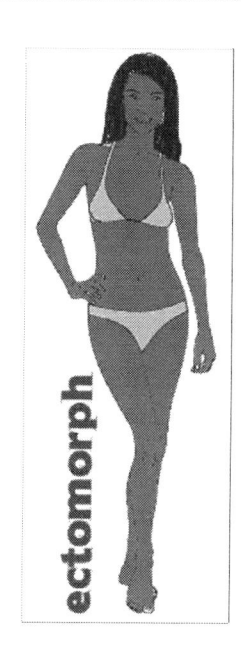

MESOMORPH BODY TYPE

Body Description

Naturally athletic, broad shoulders, narrow waist and the ability to gain muscle easily. Unlike the ectomorph, this body type doesn't have a problem gaining weight in the form of muscle or fat.

Resistance Training

Moderate to heavy weights can be used (depending on current fitness level) to maintain athletic build. A range of eight to 15 repetitions with three to four sets per muscle group will help build dense muscle tissue without giving the bulky look. If you desire less muscle, incorporate lighter weight in conjunction with a repetition range of 15 to 20.

Cardiovascular Activity

Perform cardiovascular activities (running, cycling) at least four to five days per week for at least 45 minutes. Cardiovascular activity can be performed in an interval fashion (short bursts of high intensity activity, followed by lower intensities of recovery).
Maintenance of calorie intake is important to provide sufficient energy for training and for maintaining muscle. Prolonged sessions of high intensity cardio without sufficient calories will cause body to use muscle as fuel.

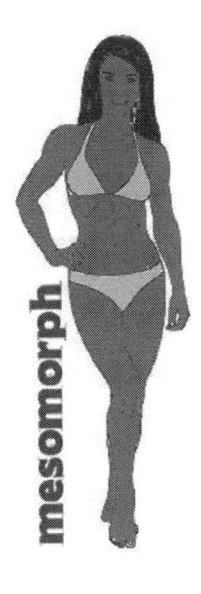

ENDOMORPH BODY TYPE

Body Description

Round, usually short in stature, carries a lot of body fat around mid-section and lower body. Slow metabolism and gains weight easily.

Resistance Training

Cardiovascular and resistance training is the key for this body type. Light to moderate weight with a repetition range of 12 to 15 with three to four sets per exercise will help tone and not build muscle. Performing activities in a circuit fashion is beneficial due to the constant state of movement throughout sets that will keep heart rate up which in return will burn more calories.

Cardiovascular Activity

Moderate to high intensity cardiovascular 45 minutes to one hour four to five days per week is recommended. Cardiovascular activities can be performed in an interval fashion (short bursts of high intensity activity, followed by lower intensities of recovery).

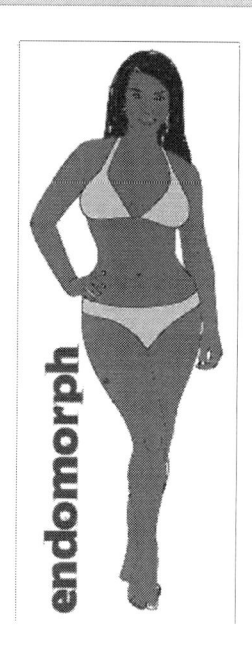

Step 2. Set Your Fitness Goals

You have discovered your body type, now it is time to learn how to set fitness training goals.

Why is it important to set goals?

Whether it is financial, marital, spiritual or physical, goal setting is an important aspect of life that keeps you focused, motivated, action-oriented and accountable. Therefore it is essential that you discover how to set fit goals. Setting fitness goals has the ability to keep you focused and motivated when you set realistic and time-sensitive goals.

Let's learn more about setting fitness goals.

Be Objective with Your Goals

Making the broad statement that you want to become fit is not concrete nor objective. You're definition of being fit needs narrowing down to a more specific or objective goal. Do you want to lose weight, gain lean muscle or improve your cardiovascular conditioning? Whatever your goal, it needs to be defined. Once your goal is defined, you can begin taking the necessary steps required to reach your desired outcome.

Measure Your Success

Goals need to be measurable. How will you determine if you are making progress if you don't know where you started? One way to determine the success of any fitness-training program is to establish a baseline of measurements. These measurements could be your body fat percentage, the amount of push-ups you can perform or how quickly you can run a specific distance. Every four to six weeks you can re-access this information to determine the progress you are making towards reaching your fitness goals.

Time is of the Essence

Setting a time frame to reach your goals is imperative to reaching your destination. You can set both short-term and long-term goals that will keep you focused and accountable.

Short-term goals are goals you want to accomplish within the next three to six months, whereas long-term goals can be accomplished within 6 months and beyond. If you are a procrastinator, setting short-term goals is very important to keep you focused and accountable. Deciding not to establish a time frame to accomplish your goal(s) threatens your chance of reaching your desired outcome.

Set Challenging Yet Realistic Goals

Finally, goals need to be challenging, yet realistic. Setting unrealistic goals perpetuates the feeling of discouragement and failure. Failure of goal attainment isn't always based on a lack of effort on your part, rather a result of setting goals that were not realistically attainable. Challenge yourself, but be realistic with your expectations.

Guidelines for Goal Setting

- Goals should be measurable.
- Goals should be challenging, yet attainable.
- Set short-term and long-term goals.
- Goals should be specific and objective.

Benefits of Setting Goals

- Greater sense of personal achievement
- Balanced life
- Increased motivation
- Improved self-confidence
- Better decision making
- Better focus
- Improved time management
- Over all self-improvement
- AND SUCCESS!

Step 3. Measure and Assess

You have discovered your body type, have learned how to set fitness goals and now it's time to discuss the importance of measurements.

Why are measurements important?

Measurements are an essential component to the success of your fitness program or weight loss program. Before starting any fitness or weight loss program, it is important to gather a baseline of information to determine a starting point and an ending point. How will you know if you're making progress towards your desired goal if you don't know where you started?

Baseline measurements can include your current weight, Body Mass Index (B.M.I), muscular endurance, flexibility and muscular strength testing. Gathering information from these sources can help you keep track of your results and every four to six weeks compare your current results to your starting baseline measurements.

Below you will discover the most common methods used to gather baseline information.

Methods of Measuring Body Composition

When you hear the words body composition, what do you think? Do you know what these words mean?

In the health and fitness world, these words are thrown around like a hot dog at a baseball game. These words are familiar to personal trainers and health care providers, but they may be foreign to you.

Body composition is a term used to describe the components that make up your body, such as lean mass, fat mass, and water. One primary goal of any fitness or weight loss program is to decrease fat mass and increase lean mass. Don't worry, you won't get bulky and look manly from gaining lean and toned muscle mass.

It is important to decrease fat mass and increase lean muscle tissue for many health reasons. Fat mass such as visceral fat which surrounds the internal organs has been linked to various health concerns, such as diabetes, hypertension and some forms of cancer.

Therefore, to make improvements in your health (and not just your appearance), you need a fitness program that focuses on gaining lean, toned muscle while at the same time losing amounts of unwanted body fat.

So how can you determine how much body fat and lean muscle mass you have?

There are several different ways that are free and painless!

I know a lot of you cringe at the thought of getting your measurements done but no worries, in the end, it will benefit your health and you will look great.

I don't want to know my numbers!

If you are one of those women who cringe at the thought of seeing measurements from your body, I want to put you at ease. These numbers don't define you; they just help to establish a starting point. I know - numbers, numbers and more numbers. You may be asking, "Do I have to?" My answer is, "YES."

I promise you, the process will be done quickly and it's painless.

We are now going to discuss the three most common and inexpensive ways to get your body composition measurements done.

FIT JEWEL

You'll never know how far you've come if you don't know where you started.

Fat Calipers

What is a fat caliper and how does it work?

A fat caliper is a small non-expensive prong-like tool used to measure subcutaneous (underneath the skin) body fat. The tester will have you stand in an upright position with arms out to your side. He or she will ask to touch your right arm and then proceed to mark designated anatomical locations (body) with a marker. The tester will then take their index finger and thumb and grasp at least two inches of your skin. The caliper will slightly grab your skin and then be released. This is a painless process that will take a few minutes to complete.

Once each spot has been located and measured, data (numbers) from the measurements are plugged into an equation to determine your percentage of body fat. Fat caliper measurements are not exact measurements, but provide you with a baseline of numbers to establish your current state of fat mass.

In order to have consistency with your measurements, have the same person administer your testing. Although each tester is required to use the same anatomical (body) locations, some testers measure differently. This difference could cause a slight variation in your numbers. You can visit your local gym or wellness center and request to have this test done for a required fee.

Below is a list of the most common anatomical locations used for measurements.

Anatomical Measuring Locations

- Triceps (back of arm)
- Supra iliac (top of hip bone)
- Sub-scapula (beneath shoulder blade)
- Biceps (middle of arm between shoulder and elbow)
- Midaxiallary- below armpit
- Sub scapula-below shoulder blade
- Thigh - midway between top of hip and knee

Girth Measurements

What is a girth measurement?

A girth measurement is a measurement that records the distance around a body part. Using this method is a non-expensive and convenient way to measure your body circumference and can be done by yourself or a trained professional. Girth measurements are sometimes used as a measure of body fat, but are not a valid predictor of this, however, can be used to measure proportionality.

How are girth measurements taken?

The only tool required to take your girth measurements is a flexible measuring tape. The person administering these measurements will use specified anatomical locations. To ensure as much accuracy as possible, the person administering the test should make sure the measuring tape isn't positioned too tight or too loose and the tape is placed in a horizontal position.

Having the tape too tight or too loose will not give you accurate measurements. Once data is collected, the administrator will use a formula to give you a total for each of your measurements. If you do not have someone to do your measurements for you, the process is simple enough to do the measurements on your own. If you measure yourself, once you gather your numbers write them down in your journal and every four to six weeks compare your numbers to see if they are changing. It is important to remember if you are building muscle tissue some numbers may increase. That is expected so do not be alarmed.

Where do you take your girth measurements?

There are several different places to take your measurements

- **Bust**: measure all the way around your bust and back starting at the nipple line.
- **Waist**: measure at the smallest point around your mid- section two inches above your navel.
- **Thigh:** measure at the largest part of the thigh, midway between hip and knee bone.
- **Calf muscle:** measure largest part midway between kneecap and ankle.
- **Arm:** measure the largest part of arm midway between shoulder joint and elbow.
- **Hips:** measure the largest part of your buttocks, place tape on thighs and measure all the way around largest part of hips.

Weight Scale

Using a weight scale is a cheap and convenient way to track your weight loss or gain. You can order an inexpensive scale online or you may visit your neighborhood Wal-Mart or Walgreens to purchase a more advanced scale that is capable of recording your body fat percentage and lean muscle mass. These advanced scales are more costly, but a great investment.

Although using a weight scale is a quick and convenient way to track your weight loss or gain, if not used in moderation, this method could lead to counterproductive behaviors.

Weighing yourself too often may discourage and distract you. It is important to remember that your body changes on a daily basis, and, as a result, your numbers may not always be consistent. Therefore, do not depend solely on the scale to dictate your progress. Although not recommended, if you decide to weigh yourself daily, do it early in the morning at the same time on a regular basis before eating or drinking anything - this is your true body weight.

Do not weigh yourself more than once a week. Healthy weight loss is a pound to two pounds per week. If you have a considerable amount of weight to lose (100lbs or more), you may lose more in the beginning but will eventually taper off. Eventually, your body will stop shedding as much body fat and you will have to re-adjust your nutrition and fitness training program to jump-start your metabolism.

Do not allow yourself to get off track by weighing yourself every day. Instead, focus your attention on energy levels, how you feel in your clothing and mental focus.

BODY MASS INDEX Measurements

What is a BMI measurement?

BMI stands for body mass index. BMI measurements are used in many health settings to help determine body fat in relation to one's height. As with any measurement, the BMI index is not an exact science.

There are many factors such as age, muscle mass and gender that are not considered in this measurement. Someone with an athletic body may register high on the BMI scale, but in all actuality have more lean mass than fat mass. Therefore, this measurement should be used with the existing knowledge that it isn't the most accurate measurement of body fat.

Although the BMI isn't an exact measure of body fat, it is a great tool to use if you want to determine whether you are at a healthy body weight for your height or at risk for certain health concerns. High BMI's (>30) have been linked to diseases such as hypertension, high cholesterol, diabetes, and obesity. Finding your BMI is a simple process that does not require expensive tools or a trained professional.

How do you calculate your BMI?

The only thing you need to calculate your BMI is a calculator and a piece of paper.

The first step in calculating your BMI is to know your current height and weight. If you do not know your current weight, find a scale and weigh yourself. If you are not aware of your height, find a measuring tape and have someone measure your height.

Follow the example below to determine your BMI by plugging in your height and weight. If you are not comfortable with numbers, you may search the World Wide Web to find a free BMI calculator to do the math for you.

Example: Amy is 150 pounds and five feet eight inches (68 inches) tall. Try this one for practice and then plug in your measurements to calculate your own BMI.

BMI Equation: Weight (kg)/Height (m) squared

1. **Determine weight in kilograms.**

    Divide pounds by 2.2. (Dividing by 2.2 converts pounds into kilograms) (Ex). 150/2.2 = 68.2 kg

2. **Determine height in meters squared.**

    First, determine ht. in cm.

    (Ex). 68 inches x 2.54 = 172.72 cm.

    Next, divide ht. in cm. by 100 to get ht. in meters. (Ex). 172.72/100 = 1.73

    Then, square ht. in meters.

    (Ex). 1.73 x 1.73 = 2.98

3. **Divide weight in kg (68.2) by height in meters squared (2.98) = 23**

4. Go to the chart below and find whether or not Amy is at a healthy BMI. If your answer is yes, then you have calculated the right answer.

CHANGING THE NORM

BMI Categories

BMI less than 18.5, falls within the "underweight" range.

BMI 18.5 to 24.9, it falls within the "normal" or "healthy weight" range.

BMI 25.0 to 29.9, it falls within the "overweight" range. Therefore, you may need to lose weight, especially if you have two or more of the risk factors for diseases associated with "overweight" range.

BMI 30.0 or higher falls within the "obese" range. Therefore, you should talk to your doctor or health care provider about weight loss options.

BMI >40, falls within the range of "morbid obesity" Therefore, you should talk to your doctor or health care provider about weight loss options and determine if you are healthy enough to exercise.

How Fit Are You?

For many women, being fit means weighing a certain amount on the scale and wearing a particular clothing size. Although having a healthy weight is important for health reasons, it doesn't define whether or not someone is fit. Being fit is a combination of muscular strength, muscular endurance, flexibility and cardiovascular endurance.

Bye, bye scale, hello pushups!

The only tools needed to determine your current level of fitness is a stopwatch, partner, and yoga mat.

Are you ready?

One-Minute Sit-Up Test:

Purpose: This test is used to determine abdominal endurance and strength. Abdominal endurance and strength are important for core stability and back support.

A. Lay on your back with knees bent. Fingers must be interlocked behind the neck and the back of hands must touch the mat. Another person holds your ankles with hands only. If you don't have someone to hold your ankles, place your feet on a firm and stable surface such as a couch.

B. On go, you or your partner will start the stop watch and you will bring your body up and bring your elbows to touch thighs. You will lower your body and return to the ground where only the upper portion of your back touches the ground. Repeat movement for one minute and then count the number of sit-ups completed. Record your numbers.

Push-Up Test (upper body strength and endurance):

Purpose: The one-minute push-up test is used to assess upper body strength and endurance.

A. Begin with the body in a push-up position. A standard push up begins with the hands and toes touching the floor, the body and legs in a straight line, feet together, arms shoulder wide apart with slight bend in elbows.

B. Keeping the back and knees straight, lower your body to a predetermined point, or until there is a 90-degree angle of the elbows, pause for a second and then return to the starting position with the arms extended without locking elbows. Repeat this action for one minute. Record your numbers.

C. If you do not have the upper body strength, perform push-ups on knees, this is considered the modified version.

3-minute Step-Up Test

Purpose: The 3-Minute Step Test measures your aerobic (cardiovascular) fitness level based on how quickly your heart rate returns to normal after exercise.

A. Before test begins, measure your resting heart rate.

Measure your resting heart rate: To do this, turn your hand over so the palm of your hand is facing upwards towards the ceiling. Locate the top of your thumb and follow your thumb until you get to the ending point of your hand. From there, using your index and middle finger, locate your radial pulse (which is located inside the hand at the base of your thumb). Don't press too hard, but gently feel for a pulse. Once you have found a pulse, set your timer and count the number of times you feel a pulse for 15 seconds and then multiply this number by four. This is your resting pulse rate. Record your numbers.

B. From there, locate a chair or bench that is at least 12 inches high. Stand in front of the bench or chair. Start the timer and slowly step on bench/chair with one foot. Then bring the other foot on bench. Use a four-step cadence, "up-up-down-down" for three minutes with a steady pace. At any time you feel out of breath or tired, stop for a moment in a standing position. Stop immediately on completion of three minutes.

C. Take pulse immediately after three minutes as explained in step A. Multiply the number of beats you count by four.

D. This number represents your heart rate after exercising.

Example: 22 beats X 4 = 88 beats per minute

The quicker your heart rate drops to its resting rate symbolizes that your cardiovascular system is becoming more conditioned. In four to six weeks, you will re-do this test and your heart rate should not get as high and you should reach your resting heart rate quicker due to your heart being more conditioned. Remember this is a starting point; you're a work in progress.

Reassess, Reassess, Reassess

Once you gather your numbers and measurements, record them and place them in your fitness journal. Four to six weeks from your original assessment date, you will want to reassess your measurements and fitness testing. You will perform the exact tests you performed above, and then compare results.

If you have noticed a positive change in numbers (ex. more strength, better cardiovascular conditioning, decreased girth measurements, BMI and Heart Rate), your fitness-training program is working and it will be time to set new fitness goals.

If you're not improving, it is recommended to re-evaluate your fitness program and motivation. During your evaluation, be honest with yourself and hold yourself accountable. Identify areas that are hindering you from reaching your goals, and from there set a realistic plan of action to reach your desired destination.

If you have not reached your goal, don't result to negative self-talk, you are working on being the best version of yourself and negative self-talk won't get you there.

Step 4. Create a Plan of Action

Let me ask you a question. Would you go on a road to trip to a particular destination without an address or directions?

Would you go on a road trip without a map or directions?

More than likely your answer is no. The same principle applies for reaching your fitness goals. It is harder to reach your destination without direction. Therefore, once you have your measurements and fitness assessment numbers recorded, it's time create a plan of attack to reach your desired fitness goals.

If your goal is to do more push-ups within a minute and build upper body strength, then a plan of action to build upper body strength is required. If you desire better cardiovascular conditioning, a cardiovascular program needs to be designed.

Whatever your goals, your plan of action needs to create the right steps to help you reach your destination.

How do you create a plan of action? Let's find out.

Create Your Plan of Attack

The first step in creating your plan of action is to find physical activities and exercise that you enjoy. If you enjoy something, you are more likely to stick with it and reach your goals easier. Working out should be an exciting time to focus on yourself and not feel tortured during the process. Therefore, it is essential to find something you enjoy doing. Many gyms offer group fitness classes including kickboxing, Zumba, spin, and boot camps. Try each one of these classes to determine which classes you enjoy most. Choose classes that are fun and are most beneficial to help you reach your fitness goal.

Fitness is about having fun. Move to your own beat. If you like to dance, just dance!

If you decide group fitness classes work for you, alternate classes to avoid overuse injuries and boredom. Overuse injuries are the result of performing the same movement patterns on a consistent basis. Constant movement patterns stress the same muscles and joints and can lead to chronic (long-term) or acute (short-term) injuries. In addition to possible overuse injuries, attending the same classes will eventually cause your body to hit a plateau and lead to limited changes in your body and cardiovascular conditioning levels.

Determine How Many Days to Exercise

Once you determine which activities you enjoy, it's time to realistically determine how many days per week you are willing to dedicate to these activities. You know your commitments more than anyone else, therefore, don't commit to more days than you can handle with your current lifestyle. If you can only do three days a week, some physical activity is better than no exercise at all. If you can't get all three days in, do what you can and don't fall into the "all or none" philosophy once you set your days of the week to exercise.

What is the "all or none" philosophy?

The "all or none" philosophy is a belief that if you miss one session of your planned activity during the week then there is no point of going for the entire week. This is a negative philosophy and mentality that can keep you from reaching your fitness goal(s). Therefore, I will once again reiterate, be realistic about the amount of days you can commit to your fitness program and some exercise is better than no exercise.

Keep Moving - It's Just Life!

If we lived in the perfect world, we could spend as much time as we wanted to be dedicated to getting fit, but unfortunately, the world and our lives aren't perfect therefore we have to be flexible with life to make sure we are getting enough physical activity in.

We get busy, emergencies and unexpected events happen, things come up that are out of our control and we sometimes get thrown off schedule, but when this happens, keep going and adapt.

Five Tips to Keep Your Body Moving When Life Happens

1. **If you can't make it to your normal scheduled class, try another class.** If you normally go to a 6:00 pm class and you're running late, try a 6:30 pm class. If there isn't one available, get creative in the gym and try a

new piece of cardio equipment or resistance training machine. Do not leave the gym without doing something healthy for yourself.

2. **Can't make it to the gym? Go for a walk.** You don't have to attend the gym to get fit. If you can't make it on a particular day, go for a walk. Walking is a great way to relieve stress and clear your mind.

3. **Keep an extra set of gym clothes and shoes in your car.** If you have to go back home to get your workout clothes, more than likely you're not going back to the gym. Therefore, always keep an extra set of gym clothes and shoes in your trunk. Consider this your emergency gym kit.

4. **You wake up late - make the most of the time you have.** If you don't wake up when the alarm goes off and all you have is 10 minutes to exercise, do something. Keep in mind doing 10 minutes of some exercise is better than no exercise at all.

5. **Your boss tells you that you have to work later than planned.** If you have to work longer than expected and you're going to miss your workout, take a brisk walk around your office building. If you have staircases in your building, take the stairs for an allotted period of time. Don't panic, life happens, just keep moving.

Step 5. Determine Your Motivation
What's Your Motivation?

The last step in beginning your fitness journey is to discover your motivation. Discovering your motivation may help you become more consistent with your fitness training program.

To discover how you are motivated, it's important to identify your motivation style.

Are you intrinsically or extrinsically motivated?

Someone who is intrinsically motivated is self-motivated and reaches goals for self-gratification and not external rewards. Intrinsically motivated people are driven by something within themselves and do not need anyone to motivate them. They set goals for themselves and are motivated to accomplish those goals without any external reward or a required cheering squad.

Then there are those who are extrinsically motivated. Extrinsically motivated people are individuals who need an external force (such as rewards or praise from other people) to motivate them. They need consistent feedback and support to feel they are doing well and without support, they are less likely to complete the task they have started. Neither one of these motivational styles are wrong, we are individuals and are driven by different motivating factors.

If you are more geared towards being extrinsically motivated, below are a few tips for you.

Tips for Extrinsically Motivated People

- Reward yourself with non-food related items when you met certain goals.

- Place a picture of what you want to look like on your fridge and in your training journal - this may help provide you with visual motivation.

- When you reach a goal, share it with someone in your support team. Sharing your success will help keep you motivated.

Steady But Gradual Progress

If you're feeling overwhelmed by all the steps you have just learned, exhale for a moment and tell yourself to focus on the process and not the outcome. Allow yourself the freedom to embrace this process without expectations of time. Your fitness journey is a jog and not a sprint, and I am confident that you will reach your destination if you give yourself time.

Chapter 22

Before You Begin

Before you make the decision to pick up a dumbbell or workout on a weight machine, it is important to understand a few key lifting techniques and training methods.

These techniques and training methods will help you avoid injury and provide you with information on how to navigate through the Iron Palace (gym) with more confidence.

Lifting Techniques

Whenever you perform an exercise (either on a machine or with free weights), there are two primary phases of movements. These phases of movement include an eccentric and concentric phase.

The concentric phase of a movement occurs when the muscle contracts or shortens. If you were executing a bicep curl, curling the weight up is the concentric phase of the movement.

The opposite, or opposing movement, is called the eccentric movement. The eccentric phase of movement involves lengthening or releasing the weight back to the starting position. If you were performing a dumbbell bicep curl and released your hand and allow the dumbbell to move downward away from your body, this would be the eccentric phase.

Each phase of movement challenges the muscles from a different level of difficulty, and one cannot be completed without the other. Therefore, it is important to only lift an amount of weight you can control during each phase of the movement. Never jeopardize form to lift heavier weight.

If an amount of weight is too heavy, choose a lighter weight. Once again I will reiterate, do not sacrifice form to lift a heavier amount of weight. Choosing to lift heavy weight in which you can't lift properly through both phases of movement can result in acute and permanent injuries.

Lifting Posture Standing

While performing any lifting movement in a standing position, feet are to be positioned slightly apart with knees slightly bent. Core or abdominals are held in tight, with shoulder blades back and chest up. Never round your back and be aware of your posture at all times.

Posture on Machines

Each machine is created to operate in a fixed range of motion meaning you can only move the machine in a predetermined movement pattern. This is beneficial in many ways, but proper posture is still required while using machines. Proper posture involves controlled movements and keeping core engaged at all times throughout the exercise.

Proper Breathing

Proper breathing consists of inhaling at the starting phase of the movement, before the beginning of the lift (concentric phase), and exhaling during the release of the weight (eccentric phase). Holding your breath while lifting can cause dizziness and create a lack of oxygen to working muscles.

FIT JEWEL

You're truly an iron sister at heart, you just don't know it yet!

Training Methods

We have discovered proper lifting techniques, now it's time to learn different resistance training methods. The following resistance training methods are the most common and most applicable.

Split Training

Split training is a term used to identify how each muscle group is divided and trained. Using the split training method ensures each muscle group is trained on a consistent basis, to avoid muscular imbalances and muscular injuries from under and overdeveloped muscles.

How do you create a split training routine that is right for you?

To create your individualized split, determine how many days a week you can dedicate to resistance training. Once you have completed this task, decide which muscle groups you want to train together or by themselves (ex. Biceps and Triceps, Back and Chest). Some research suggests training your muscles in a push/pull fashion, but you make the decision. This method is believed to create muscular balances if done properly.

Training in a push/pull fashion involves training muscles that allow you to perform pushing and pulling movements within the same training session. Doing a push-up is considered a pushing movement (which uses your chest muscles), followed by seated dumbbells rows (which is a pulling movement) which work the back muscles.

Split training is designed based on individual preference, and your split may not mirror your girlfriends. Once you create your split schedule, it does not have to be set in stone. Changing the muscle groups and the days, you train them are beneficial both mentally and physically.

Possible Disadvantage of the Split Training Method

Although split training is a great training method, it is important to consider your current level of fitness before you create your split training routine.

Spilt training typically focuses on training one or two body parts per training session. Typically, the volume or the number of sets and repetitions you perform using this training method places more stress on your muscles. Placing a great amount of stress on untrained muscles can lead to excessive soreness and injuries. Therefore, if you are not at a training level where you can perform split training, full body training may be more advantageous for you.

Advantages of Split Training

A benefit of split training for seasoned lifters is the ability to train a weak muscle group(s). With this method of training, you can focus on that particular group during your training session and perform more sets which can assist in strengthening your weaker muscle groups.

Example of Split Training

Monday:	Biceps/Triceps/Abs
Tuesday:	Chest/Back
Wednesday:	Off
Thursday:	Shoulders/Abs
Friday:	Legs/Abs
Saturday:	Off

Full Body Training

As the name states, full body training is a method that targets each major muscle group within one training session. Full body training is a great method for beginners and for individuals who do not have enough time to devote to a split training regimen.

Full body training targets each muscle group, but it doesn't stress each individual muscle group as efficiently as split training. When you are doing a full body training session, you are typically performing one or two exercises per muscle group. This will help you tone, but to experience continual muscle growth, you will eventually need to stress each muscle group beyond full body training.

Example of Full Body Training

2 sets per exercise, 12 to 15 repetitions

	Set 1	Set 2
Legs	Lunges	Squats
Biceps	Bicep Curls	Hammer Curls
Triceps	Triceps Extensions	Triceps Kickbacks
Shoulders	Lateral Shoulder Raises	Front Shoulder Raises
Back	One-arm Rows	Seated Rows
Abs	Crunches	Leg Lifts

Super Setting

Super setting requires performing one exercise for a primary muscle group, followed immediately by performing an exercise for its opposing muscle group. Super setting keeps your muscles in balance due to the consistency of training both sides of your muscle group.

Super setting will cut back on gym time and allow the body to maintain balance within each muscle group.

Example of Super Setting

Biceps/Triceps (bicep curls followed immediately by triceps extensions)

Back/Chest (lat pull downs, followed immediately by pushups)

Quads/Hamstrings (leg extensions, followed immediately by hamstring curls)

Giant Set

Performing a giant set requires choosing a particular muscle group and choosing four to five different exercises for that particular group.

After choosing your exercises, perform each exercise in a circuit fashion, moving from one exercise to another without rest until the set is complete.

Create your giant set based on your current fitness level. You can begin with two to three different exercises, and then progressively increase the amount of exercises as you become stronger and better conditioned.

Example of a Giant Set

Muscle Group: Shoulders

Lateral shoulder raises	10 repetitions
Front shoulder raises	10 repetitions
Seated shoulder press	10 repetitions
Rear deltoid raises	10 repetitions

Circuit Training

Circuit training involves performing a group of exercises in a continuous fashion, and not reaching a stopping point until each exercise is completed.

Circuit training is believed to be an effective training method for people who are short on time and desire more cardiovascular conditioning.

Cardiovascular conditioning is a result of a continually elevated heart rate throughout the circuit.

Example of Circuit Training

Remember to perform each exercise in a continual fashion before you reach a state of rest.

CHANGING THE NORM

Stationary lunges	12 repetitions
Standing bicep curls	12 repetitions
Triceps kickbacks	12 repetitions
Standing shoulder press	12 repetitions
Modified pushups	8-10 repetitions
Crunches	12 repetitions

Interval Training

Interval training involves performing short periods of high-intensity exercise followed immediately by the same activity at a lower intensity.

Studies show interval training burns more calories than regular steady state (performing exercise at the same pace over a period of time) physical activities.

Intervals can be created during any activity.

Example of Interval Training

An example of interval training would be sprinting on the treadmill at a 6.9 speed for 30 seconds followed by jogging at a speed of 4.0 for one minute. Repeat interval five times)

Determine Your Sets, Repetitions, and Weight

One of the most common questions women have when it comes to resistance training is, "How much weight should I lift to reach my goals?"

The amount of weight you lift is based on your fitness goals. If you desire to build toned, lean muscles, you will perform exercises with light weight five to 15 pounds) within a repetition range of 15 to 20 repetitions while performing at least three sets of each exercise.

If your goal is to build an athletic body with more dense muscle tissue, you will lift heavier weight (15 pounds or more) within a range of eight to 15 repetitions performing at least 4-5 sets of each exercise.

As a rule of thumb, the heavier weight you use, the fewer repetitions you will perform. This builds strength and muscle density.

The lighter weight you use, the higher repetitions you will perform. This will create lean, toned muscles.

Wait I Still Have Questions!

Walking into a room full of men with bulging biceps can leave you doubting the choice you have made to start a resistance training program, but equipping yourself with the proper armor before you enter the Iron Palace will give you more confidence and the ability to freely navigate your way through.

Entering the Iron Palace may seem intimidating right now, but below you will discover answers to the most frequently asked questions from women regarding resistance and cardiovascular training. Knowing the answers to these questions may help you feel more confident when you enter the Iron Palace.

FAQs Regarding Resistance and Cardiovascular Training

Q. HOW MANY DAYS A WEEK SHOULD I LIFT?

A. It is recommended that beginners start with two to three days per week performing total body workouts or using machines. The beginning of your fitness training program should be gradual, with an emphasis on technique or lifting form. Training too frequently or intensely at this stage of your fitness-training program could lead to injuries and early burn out.

Intermediate and advanced trainees can train four to five days per week, allowing at least 48 hours of rest per muscle group. If you are in a training rut, revamp your entire fitness training program by overloading your body with more repetitions, heavier weight, different exercises, and less rest time in between sets.

A rule of thumb - if you have been using the same fitness training program for more than six weeks, it is time to update your program.

Q. MACHINES OR FREE WEIGHTS?

A. Both. Using a combination of machines and free weights can assist you in reaching your fitness goals.

CHANGING THE NORM

Machines

Machines are great for beginners, they are easy to operate and provide step-by-step instructions. Most machines provide pictorials to identify which muscle groups are used during the execution of the movement. Machines are created to move in a fixed range of motion that prevents improper form and this is beneficial to individuals who aren't experienced with resistance training. Using machines does not require a high level of coordination, balance or strength for beginners.

Free Weights

Using free weights requires proper knowledge of form in order to execute each desired exercise. Using free weights also requires balance, coordination and core strength. Free weights engage more muscular activity than using machines and can challenge the body in a different manner than machines. More muscle engagement means more calories burned. More calories burned means a more lean and toned body.

Q. HOW MUCH WEIGHT SHOULD I LIFT?

A. Beginners

Beginners are recommended to find an amount of weight that will allow them to perform 12 to 15 repetitions safely throughout an entire range of movement. When reaching the 15th repetition if the weight is still challenging to lift, stay with that amount of weight. Once you reach a point where the weight is no longer challenging, make small increases in weight. You can progress from 5 lbs. to 8 lbs. then to 10 lbs. This process is known as progressive resistance training.

Intermediate and Advanced Trainees

Select an amount of weight heavy enough that will allow you to execute eight to 15 repetitions with proper form. If you reach your 15th repetition and the weight is not challenging, increase the weight by 5 lbs.

Q. HOW MANY REPETITIONS DO I PERFORM?

A. The number of repetitions performed for any exercise is determined by your fitness goals.

For Power Moves
- 2 to 3 repetitions
- Heavy weight
- This will help athletes develop power and explosiveness.

For Muscular Strength
- 8 to 15 repetitions
- Moderate to heavy weight
- This will help build lean and dense muscle tissue.

For Muscular Endurance
- 15 to 20 repetitions
- Light weight
- This will help tone lean muscles

Q. HOW MUCH CARDIO SHOULD I DO?

A. Cardiovascular activity should be a part of every person's fitness training program, but shouldn't be the only method used to get fit. Cardiovascular activities not only burn body fat, they keep your heart (the most important muscle in your body) in shape, but they don't build lean muscles.

According to The American College of Sports Medicine and the American Heart Association, perform at least 60 minutes of moderate to vigorous physical activity most days of the week.

However, the specific amount of cardio you need varies from person to person and depends on the following factors:
- Daily caloric intake
- Exercise intensity and frequency
- Your metabolic rate (rate of substance breakdown)
- Your current fitness level (sedentary individuals will require a gradual increase in cardiovascular activities)
- Your body fat percentage

- Your current weight
- Your fitness goals

Beginners

Perform at least 25 to 30 minutes of light-to-moderate intensity cardiovascular activities most days of the week. Gradually progress where you can perform 35 to 45 minutes of continuous cardiovascular activities as your heart and lungs become more conditioned.

Intermediate and Advanced

Perform at least 40 minutes to one hour, including intervals.

Q. WHAT IS A HEART RATE?

A. Heart rate is the number of beats the heart takes within one minute. There is a direct correlation between heart rate and workload (work performed). As workload or intensity increases, heart rate will increase. To keep track of your heart rate, you may purchase a heart rate monitor. Wearing a heart rate monitor will help gauge your intensity levels at all times.

Q. HOW DO I FIND MY PULSE RATE TO DETERMINE HOW INTENSE I AM EXERCISING?

A. You can determine your pulse rate by using your radial pulse (arm). In order to locate your radial pulse, turn your hand over with thumb turned in an outward position. Start at tip of thumb and go all the way to the base of your thumb and move about half an inch from base of thumb using index and middle fingers and search for a pulse.

Once pulse is located, count the number of heart beats for 10 seconds. Multiply this number by six. This number will give you your heart rate.

Setting a target heart rate will give you an intensity level to reach for while exercising.

Know Your Numbers

The table below shows estimated target heart rates for different ages. In the age category closest to yours, read across to find your target heart rate. Your maximum heart rate is about 220 minus your age. The figures are averages, so use them as general guidelines.

Age	Target HR Zone, 50-85%	Average Maximum Heart Rate, 100%
20 years	100-170 beats per minute	200 beats per minute
30 years	95-162 beats per minute	190 beats per minute
35 years	93-157 beats per minute	185 beats per minute
40 years	90-153 beats per minute	180 beats per minute
45 years	88-149 beats per minute	175 beats per minute
50 years	85-145 beats per minute	170 beats per minute
55 years	83-140 beats per minute	165 beats per minute
60 years	80-136 beats per minute	160 beats per minute
65 years	78-132 beats per minute	155 beats per minute
70 years	75-128 beats per minute	150 beats per minute

Q. IN WHAT ORDER SHOULD I PERFORM MY EXERCISES?

A. If you are training to become powerful, power moves are performed first in your workout program. Power moves require lifting heavy amounts of weight that fatigue your neuromuscular system and should not be performed when you are fatigued. Lifting heavy amounts of weight when you are fatigued can lead to permanent injuries. Therefore all power moves should occur at the beginning of your fitness routine (ex. Plyometrics)

Next, you will want to perform exercises that require the use of larger muscles (legs, chest, back) or multi-joint exercises. These exercises require more energy to perform, therefore, should be done before performing single-joint exercises which require less effort.

Last to be performed are smaller or single-joint exercises (shoulders, triceps, biceps). To avoid fatigue, do not train smaller muscles first. Training your smaller muscle groups first will cause you to fatigue quicker and lead to a less-than-optimal training session for your larger muscle groups.

CHANGING THE NORM

Q. HOW MUCH REST TIME SHOULD I TAKE IN BETWEEN SETS?

A. The amount of rest time taken in between sets is determined by the amount of weight used and the intensity level at which you perform the exercise. Performing powerful and explosive movements may require 3-5 minutes of rest. This amount of rest time is needed to produce more energy and allows your neurological system time to recuperate.

For lower intensity exercises, rest for 30-90 seconds and no longer.

Q. HOW MUCH REST TIME SHOULD I TAKE OFF BETWEEN WORKOUT SESSIONS?

A. Resistance training involves breaking down muscle fibers (muscle tissue) that result in muscular soreness referred to as D.O.M.S. (Delayed Onset Muscle Soreness). The body naturally repairs these micro tears during rest. Therefore, not getting the proper amount of rest can lead to overtraining, diminishes in strength and a weakened immune system and fatigue.

Therefore, it is recommended to allow at least 48 hours of rest time between the training of each muscle group. If you are afraid to take a complete day off, you may take part in activities called active rest. During active rest, you are performing more leisure-based activities such as walking the dog, gardening or maybe going for a casual walk.

Below are signs of training burnout and overtraining. Familiarize yourself with these signs and be mindful that more isn't always better!

Signs of Burnout or Overtraining

- Weakened immune system (more susceptible to infections)
- Decrease in motivation
- Excessive muscle soreness
- Irritability
- Decreases in strength

CHANGING THE NORM

Q. CAN MUSCLE TURN INTO FAT?

A. No, muscle and fat are two separate types of tissue. One cannot convert into the other.

When muscle tissue is not stressed by lifting adequate amounts of weight (resistance), the muscles atrophy (become smaller).

When a person gains fat weight, it is not a result of muscle tissue turning into fat; it is a result of an increase in size of their fat cells.

Q. SHOULD I DO CARDIO OR WEIGHTS?

A. To create a strong, lean and toned physique you need to incorporate both.

To all of my resistance training enthusiasts, resistance training is great for building lean muscle tissue, but without cardiovascular activity, that six pack you have been working so hard to create may not be seen. Body fat can threaten to hide your hard-earned muscle and one of the ways you can show off what you have worked hard for is to incorporate cardiovascular activities into your regular fitness training sessions along with clean eating.

To my cardio queens, if the only thing you do is cardio, I want to encourage you to step into the Iron Palace and begin a resistance training program. Cardiovascular activities will change your size, but it will not change the shape of your body. Resistance training will help build a toned, calorie-burning machine.

Chapter 23

Learn The Principles and Terminology

Applying the following principles will provide you with an understanding of weight lifting terminology and principles.

You are your sister's keeper therefore, make sure you share this information with your girlfriends and invite them to the gym the next time you go!

Principle of Individual Differences - Everyone has a different genetic makeup and different training needs. Your fitness training program needs to be designed around your individuality. Your friend's training program may not work for you.

Principle of Adaptation - The body is a dynamic creation that changes when constant external (resistance training/weights) forces are applied. In order for your body to grow, continue to challenge your body with more repetitions, sets and volume of training.

Principle of Specificity - The only way to master a particular exercise or skill is to execute that particular exercise or skill on a regular basis. Specificity training is a very big principle in the athletic world. In order for a swimmer to become better at swimming, he/she has to swim. If you want to become great at a particular exercise, perform that exercise on a regular basis and your body will eventually adapt.

Principle of Progression - Placing too much stress or load on your body in a short period of time can lead to injuries. Therefore, gradually increase the amount of weight and intensity of each exercise you perform. Doing this will prevent excessive soreness, over training and mental burnout.

Principle of Use/Disuse - It is a cliché, but it is true. "If you don't use it, you lose it." When muscles are under consistent tension or stress, they adapt and grow. This process is called hypertrophy.

When muscles are not stressed, they become smaller and weaker. A process called atrophy. If you incorporate a resistance training program for a period of time, then stop for a longer period of time, your muscles will atrophy (become smaller). No stress means no growth.

Principle of Overload - Once the body adapts to a stress or load, it has to be challenged with more stress or load. Continuing to perform the same exercises, sets, repetitions and rest time does not challenge the body enough to force it to change. You have to overload your body and there is no way around this principle.

Abduction - movement away from the midline of the body (e.g. doing seated abductions on a machine). In this exercise, you bring your legs from an inward position to an outward position.

Adduction – movement towards the midline of the body e.g. doing seated adductions on a machine). In this exercise, you bring your legs from an outward position to an inward position.

Atrophy - loss of muscle due to lack of training stimulus.

Cardiovascular - pertains to your heart, veins and arteries.

Concentric - upward or contraction phase of a movement/muscle shortens (muscle contracts).

Dorsi Flexion - pointing toes upward towards the ceiling.

Eccentric - downward or negative phase of a movement/muscle lengthens (muscle relaxes).

Elbow extension - movement resulting in an increase of the elbow joint (triceps extension) of the body. These planes of motion allow the body to move in a certain direction and help identify movements of particular joints.

Elbow flexion - movement resulting in a decrease of the elbow joint (performing a bicep curl).

Extension - increases the angle of a joint (performing leg extensions is an example of knee extension).

Flexibility - range of motion around a joint.

Flexion - decreases the angle of a joint (performing a bicep curls is an example of elbow flexion).

Hyperextend - to go beyond a point or distance.

Hypertrophy - muscular growth due to training stimulus.

Lateral - side movement (e.g. lateral shoulder raises).

Muscular Endurance - the ability to continually exert force against a resistance.

Maximum heart rate - the highest number of times your heart beats in one minute.

Muscular Strength - the ability to exert a maximal amount of force against resistance.

Plantar Flexion - pointing toes downward.

Primary muscle - intended targeted muscle you want to train (when performing bicep curls, primary muscle is the bicep).

Respiratory - pertains to your lungs.

Repetition - repeated movement of a particular exercise.

Rotation - side-to-side or left-to-right movement of the trunk (top part of body) (e.g. performing Russian Twists) or neck.

Set - designated amount of repetitions.

Chapter 24

Social Hour is Over

This Isn't Club Talk

Being around like-minded fitness enthusiasts can help you reach your fitness goals and possibly lead you to make lifetime friendships.

However, working out at the gym can become a place where you can get distracted from reaching your fitness goals.

Distracted, who me?

As women, many of us have one thing in common, we love to socialize!

Yes, many of us are social butterflies. This can be a great thing at the right time and right place, however, it is not social hour when you walk through the gym doors. You are there to train and focus on your fitness goals.

Does this mean you have to be unfriendly and non-sociable?

Not at all, but it does mean that 90 percent of your time shouldn't be spent talking. Talking and not working out will prevent you from reaching your fitness goals. If you enjoy chatting, have your talks during your cool down and stretching.

Before we continue, let me share a pet peeve of mine.

If you are new to the gym, you may not be able to relate to this, but if you're a "gymette," you will know exactly what I mean. Let me paint the picture for you.

Please Don't Distract Me!

It has been a long day at work and all you can think about is getting to the gym and having a grueling workout. OK, maybe you don't enjoy the grueling aspect of training, but follow me anyway. You rush to the gym and can't wait for some alone time.

You change into your training gear and are ready to train. You walk out into the Iron Palace and you begin your warm up. You have your music on the right song and you are starting to feel your body's core temperature increase. Ten minutes of a general warm up and you are ready to attack the IRON.

CHANGING THE NORM

You get your gloves on and all you can think about is the feeling of iron held in your hands. You scope out your weapon of mass destruction and head in that direction. On the way there you have the eye of the tiger and all of a sudden someone stops and says "Hi, how are you?" You do not want to lose your focus and at the same time, you don't want to be rude. You say, "I'm great thanks." Another question comes. "So how is work?" You think, "Oh no if I do not walk away more questions are going to follow."

Sure enough, you try to walk off and the person keeps talking. You are cooling down and someone has taken the equipment you wanted to use. Can you say frustrated? If you are laughing right about now, you know exactly what I am talking about.

The gym is a great place to meet people, but keep in mind - it isn't social hour when you are there. It's great to talk but make your conversations polite and brief. Don't spend the majority of your time talking with friends or associates. If you do, you are losing time that could be invested in you transforming your body. How can you build a fit body if you spend the majority of your time talking?

A rule of thumb to keep in mind is - time spent in the gym does not automatically mean time spent on training. I frequently meet women who share that their fitness program just isn't working. When I ask them if they are in the gym for social hour or to train, many of the responses correspond with the latter.

If you are talking more than you're working, more than likely your mind is not focused on exercising. Therefore, here's your new mantra. "When it's time to train, it's time to train." Save the talking for cardio time.

Avoid Wasting Gym Time

- ✓ **Talk during rest time:** It is great having friends at the gym, but keep in mind you are there to train and not have social hour. Talk during your rest time between sets, but stay focused on why you're there.
- ✓ **Plan ahead of time:** Have a plan of action before you hit the gym. Know which muscle(s) you are going to train and what exercises you are going to do before you arrive. Having a plan of attack will keep you from wondering around not sure of what to do.

- ✓ **Don't wait around:** If a machine you want is occupied, politely ask the individual when they are going to be finished. Do not waste time waiting for a particular machine. Do another exercise and come back at a later time.

- ✓ **Perform exercises in a circuit fashion**: A circuit involves choosing at least four different exercises for the entire body, and performing one exercise then immediately performing another without reaching a state of rest until all exercises are complete. Training in this fashion will keep your heart rate up and decrease gym time.

- ✓ **Double check your gym bag:** Before leaving home, double check your gym bag to make sure you have socks, gym shoes, training clothes and hair ties. This will help you from having to go back home or stop at the store to purchase these items. This saves time and money.

- ✓ **Bring your own water:** Have enough water to avoid frequent trips to the water fountain. Carry a large container to hold water instead of little 16 oz. bottles that require many refills.

- ✓ **Fuel up**: Eat a source of protein and complex carbohydrate at least one hour before your workout. Not having enough fuel can hinder your workout and prevent you from fully exerting yourself.

FIT JEWEL

Talk during your rest time between sets, but stay focused on why you're there.

Chapter 25

Gym Etiquette 101

If you are a newcomer to the gym, this class will be new to you.

If you are a seasoned gym veteran, this will be a refresher course.

After spending many years in the gym, you become aware of what is acceptable and what is not.

There are spoken and unspoken rules at the gym and now that you are going to be a part of this culture, it is important you learn proper gym etiquette.

The rules are as follows:

Rule 1: Don't sit in sauna without clothes

We are all women, but there is something very awkward about having someone in the nude right in front of you doing things that most people would consider private. Being comfortable in your own skin is great, but be aware there are other people who may not feel comfortable with you walking around in the nude. Embrace your body, but please put a towel on.

FIT JEWEL

There are spoken and unspoken rules at the gym – it's important to learn gym etiquette!

Rule 2: Don't use bathroom stalls to change clothes

The bathroom should be used just for what is has been created for. If you are uncomfortable changing in front of other people it's understandable, but please don't change in the bathroom. Doing this holds the lineup when other people need to use the restroom. Please be considerate and go into the shower area or other private designated area and change. Normally there is more space in these areas, and you will not hold up the restrooms.

Rule 3: No perfume overload

There is a time and place for everything, but wearing heavy amounts of perfume to the gym is definitely not the right time or place. Instead of using heavy perfumes that may affect other people, try a light body spray.

Rule 4: No machine hoarding

Depending on the time of day, the gym can become overly crowded. If this is the case, you may have to share equipment with other people. If this happens, be open and willing to share. If you are working on a machine and taking a rest, allow someone else to use the machine during your rest time. Be friendly and respectful to everyone and if you are not using a machine, do not sit and talk on the machine. This hinders other people from using the machine.

Rule 5: Do not interrupt

It is an unspoken rule, but a very important one. Do not interrupt someone during a set. If someone is in the middle of lifting weights or performing an exercise, wait until they are done before you interrupt them. It is rude and can break someone's focus if you speak to them while they are executing a movement. If you need to ask a question, wait until that person has completed with their set. If they are not finished, do not stand and wait. Walk away and come back when they are finished.

Rule 6: No cell phone on gym floor

Cell phones can be a huge distraction to you and others. Talking on the phone while working out can be dangerous and annoying to others around you. If you need to talk, find a quiet place in the gym to excuse yourself. Some gyms do not allow members to talk on cell phones. If you train at a gym that has this rule, respect this rule and set an example to others.

If you are allowed to use your cell phone, keep in mind that other people come to the gym to de-stress and loud conversations on your cell phone can be disturbing.

Rule 7: Make a mess, clean your mess

It is unhealthy and very inconsiderate to leave your sweat on machines, mats or other equipment. Hundreds of people train at the gym and leave behind bacteria and certain viruses on a daily basis. To help prevent the spread of germs and avoid getting sick, wipe down your equipment after each use. If there isn't any cleaner available, don't be afraid to ask gym staff to provide you with some antibacterial cleaner.

CHANGING THE NORM

Prevent the Spread of Harmful Bacteria

- Wash hands before and after using the restroom.
- Wipe machines off before use and immediately afterward.
- If you are sick, stay at home.
- If you sneeze, do so towards the inside of your elbow. This will keep you from using your hands and then touching equipment.
- If you perspire heavily, bring a towel to keep your surrounding area clean.
- If your gym is out of sanitizer, nicely request to have the bottles refilled and spray equipment after every use.
- If you are using a mat to exercise, please be polite and clean it and then put it back when you are done. No one wants to search for a mat or lie on a mat that is covered in sweat.
- Cover any open cuts or wounds. Bacteria can get into open areas and cause infection.
- Do not place hands around your eyes or mouth during your workout.
- Wash hands before leaving the gym. Although the gym is a place to get fit and healthy, there's a lot of unwanted bacteria lurking around.

Talking on your cell phone while others are working out can be distracting to them and it can also hinder you from effectively focusing on your workout. Allow this time to be only for emergency calls. Besides, this is time dedicated for yourself, why let others interrupt you?

Chapter 26

Cardio Fit

Are You the Queen of Cardio?

For many women, performing endless hours of cardio has become the solution to weight loss and getting into shape.

Although cardio can assist you in losing weight, doing endless hours of cardio will not ultimately get your body into the best shape.

You may have been taught that this is the only way to reach your fitness and weight loss goals, but I would like to share a better way to help you reap more benefits from doing less cardio.

How does that sound?

Do Less and Reap More

Although steady state (exercising at same intensity level for a period of time) cardio has its benefits, interval training can be more beneficial and require less time.

Studies have shown that performing 15-20 minutes of interval training can burn more calories than performing 40-45 minutes of steady state cardio if done at the appropriate intensity level. Therefore, why spend endless hours doing steady state cardio, when you can spend less time and gain more results by doing interval training?

Interval What?

What is interval training?

Interval training consists of performing short bursts of high-intensity activity followed by short periods of lower intensity activity. You can create an interval on any piece of cardio equipment, with running or walking.

An example of a jog/sprint interval could consist of sprinting to a certain landmark (such as a mailbox) and then jogging to another landmark (such as a stop sign).

CHANGING THE NORM

The intensity of your high bursts is based on your current level of fitness and as with any physical activity, interval training should be done in moderation and safely. Interval training requires higher bursts of movements, and if done too fast for beginners could result in injuries.

FIT JEWEL

Doing endless hours of cardio will not ultimately get your body into the best shape.

Therefore, it is recommended beginners perform intervals one to two times per week at the beginning of your fitness program and increase the frequency as your cardiovascular condition improves.

For individuals who are intermediate or advanced, perform intervals three to four days per week allowing yourself at least 48 hours of rest per week. Too much of any good thing is bad for you.

How Do You Create an Interval?

Determine your current fitness level and cardiovascular conditioning (beginner, intermediate or advanced).

Determine how much cardio you desire to perform.

Choose a machine(s), or decide if you want to perform walking or running intervals.

Based on your fitness level, create an interval for a desired amount of time.

The amount of time you rest is based on the intensity of activity (e.g., you can sprint on the treadmill for 20 seconds and then walk for 30 seconds).

The higher the intensity of each activity, typically the longer the rest/recovery time (e.g., If you sprint for 30 seconds you may need 45 seconds to one minute to recover by jogging or walking at a slower pace).

Interval Tip: Most cardio machines have programmed intervals. If you are not sure how to use your gym equipment, do not be afraid to ask for assistance.

Intensity Please!

To get the most bang for your buck, make sure you are putting in the right amount of INTENSITY into your intervals.

CHANGING THE NORM

Intensity is the amount of effort you put into your exercise and one way to determine your effort is to use the R.P.E. (Rate of Perceived Exertion) scale.

What is the R.P.E. scale?

The R.P.E. is a subjective scale using the numbers zero through ten to rank your intensity (effort put into activity) during your physical activity.

By learning this scale, you can determine if you are putting enough effort into your interval sessions. This scale can be used for your resistance training routine as well.

R.P.E. SCALE	
0	NOTHING AT ALL
1	VERY LIGHT
2	FAIRLY LIGHT
3	MODERATE
4	SOMEWHAT HARD
5	HARD
6	
7	VERY HARD
8	
9	
10	VERY HARD (MAXIMAL Intensity)

Are You Tired of The Same Old Thing?

Doing cardio on a treadmill or elliptical can eventually become boring and cause overuse injuries due to performing the same movement patterns on a regular basis.

Besides, don't you get tired of the same old thing? Then, why not get creative with your cardio?

It's time to think outside the box and try the following cardio blast program.

This cardio blast routine will challenge your body by giving your mind a break from the monotony of your daily grind on the treadmill.

Items needed: Jump rope, bench or stable chair and medicine ball

CHANGING THE NORM

Step 1: Gather needed items: Jump rope, bench or stable chair, medicine ball, your body.

Step 2: Identify your skill level (beginner, intermediate or advanced) and follow recommended sets and repetitions.

Step 3: Perform each exercise. At any point, adjust sets and repetitions according to your skill level and personal difficulty.

The following exercises are performed in a circuit fashion. Perform one exercise then move immediately to the next exercise without resting. Complete each exercise and then come to a state of rest.

General Warm-Up: Perform five to 10 minutes of light activity, such as jogging in place or walking on a treadmill.

Jump Rope: Body standing straight with a slight bend in knees. Hold rope lightly in hands. Turn rope, maintain soft bend in knees, stay on the base of feet. Do not pound feet on the ground.

Step Ups: Stand in front of chair or bench with feet slightly apart and bend in knees. Keep upper body straight with core tight, arms by side. Slowly step up on bench with left foot, then right foot. Step back with opposite foot, until both feet are on ground, then repeat.

Med Ball Throw Downs: While standing straight, position med ball chest level using both hands. With a slight bend in the knees, move body in an upward movement, bringing the ball over your head and then throwing the ball toward the ground. Let the ball rebound, then catch. Repeat movement.

Line Hops: Create an imaginary line on the surface you are using. Stand behind an imaginary line. While standing straight with slight bend in knees, jump forward over line, then jump back over the same line in the opposite direction. Keep a soft bend in your knees throughout the entire movement. Repeat.

Lateral Hops: Create an imaginary line on the surface you are using. Stand on the side of the imaginary line. While standing straight with slight bend in knees, jump over line in a lateral (side movement), then jump back over same line in opposite direction. Keep a soft bend in knees throughout entire movement. Repeat.

Beginners: Rest at least one minute, 30 seconds after the circuit is complete.

Sets	Performance Time	Repetitions
2-3	20-25 seconds	10-12

*Jump rope for 20 to 30 seconds

Intermediate: Rest one minute after entire circuit is complete.

Sets	Performance Time	Repetitions
3-4	25-40 seconds	15-20

* Jump rope for 30 to 45 seconds

Advanced: Rest 30 to 45 seconds after entire circuit is complete.

Sets	Performance Time	Repetitions
5-6	45 seconds – 1 minute	25-30

*Jump rope for 1 minute - 1 minute, 15 seconds

If or when you use cardio machines at the gym, please use the following guidelines to get the most out of your cardio sessions.

Cardio Guidelines

Do not lean on cardio machines: The handles that are provided on each cardio machine are not created for you to lean on. At all times keep body in an upright position with core tight. Leaning on the cardio machine takes away the effectiveness of the exercise by allowing the machines to support your body. Get the most out of every session and don't cheat yourself.

Pay Attention: If you are going to read while doing cardio, make sure your intensity level is sufficient enough to burn calories. Many people read and do not exert enough effort into their cardio. If you want to read, try using the recumbent bike where you can sit and read but still pedal fast.

Get Creative: Using the same cardio machines repeatedly can cause overuse injuries and mental burnout. It is good to mix up your cardio. If you like the bike, why not try adding the elliptical or the stair stepper?

CHANGING THE NORM

Try Cardio Intervals: Why spend an hour walking slowly on the treadmill when you can spend 30 to 35 minutes doing intervals and burn more calories? Don't be afraid to try new things - it will shock your body and jump start your metabolism.

Sister to Sister Tip: Doing Long Hours Of Cardio Won't Help You Get The Body You Want!

Chapter 27

Stretching Essentials

There are numerous benefits to stretching, such as increased range of motion, decreased muscle stiffness and prevention of certain injuries.

With so many benefits, stretching should be performed most days of the week following all physical activity.

Choosing not to stretch on a regular basis can hinder your range of motion and lead to injuries.

Therefore, let's learn some basics of proper stretching.

What is range of motion (ROM)?

Range of motion is the pain-free movement around a joint(s). The key word is pain-free. As we age, we begin to experience stiffness of our joints and movements become painful as a result of not stretching on a regular basis. Chronic stiffness can lead to limited range of motion, which can lead to improper body mechanics and injuries.

Therefore, to avoid these issues, use the following guidelines to stretching and make stretching a regular part of your fitness training program.

Stretching Guidelines

Never stretch a cold muscle. Imagine placing a rubber band in the freezer for a period of time and then attempting to stretch it. It will not be as pliable cold as it would be at room temperature. Your muscles, ligaments, and tendons are similar to a rubber band. The warmer they become, the more pliable they will be. This elasticity will help prevent injuries and increase your range of motion.

Stretch after your workout before complete cool down. Muscles need to have the ability to contract and produce force, therefore stretching too much before your workout could result in less force generated during your lifting. Stretching is used to relax and elongate the muscles, and over stretching before resistance training may prevent optimal performance. To avoid this, stretch before you reach a cooldown state immediately after your training session.

CHANGING THE NORM

Never bounce. Your body has protective mechanisms which detect the length and force of a stretch. If you stretch your muscles too fast or too far, the body will respond by contracting the muscles. Do not force your body to go beyond its normal range of motion by bouncing or forcing yourself into a stretched position. Forcing your body to go beyond this point can lead to injuries.

Stretch at least three days per week. Regular stretching will provide a greater range of motion to perform Activities of Daily Living (ADLs) such as grocery shopping, gardening, and cleaning. Being flexible will, also, help you with sports-related performances and lessen chances of injury.

Follow the F.I.T.T. Model for Stretching

The F.I.T.T. model below teaches you the frequency, intensity, type, and time for stretching.

Frequency: At least three days per week, preferably daily and after all physical activity

Intensity: Slow, controlled and not forced. Slowly elongate muscle with low level of force

Type: At least four to five stretches per major muscle groups (legs, arms, chest, back)

Time: 15 to 30 second holds (static stretching)

The following stretches can be performed after each workout. Remember each stretching guideline and do not force your body beyond its normal range of motion.

Upper Body Stretches
(Shoulders, Back, Triceps, Chest, Biceps)

Triceps Stretch (standing)

Stand in an upright position with a slight bend in knees. Raise your arm over your head and bend your elbow all the way so your hand is behind your neck. Use your opposite arm to stabilize your elbow. Hold for 15to 30 seconds. Repeat three to five times and then perform stretch on the opposite side.

Triceps Stretch (sitting)

Sit in a chair with body in an upright position, core tight and shoulders back. Raise your arm over your head and bend your elbow all the way so your hand is behind your neck. Use your opposite arm to stabilize your elbow. Hold for 15 to 30 seconds. Repeat three to five times and then perform stretch on the opposite side.

Shoulder Rolls

Begin sitting or standing with your arms at your sides. Shrug your shoulders up. While your shoulders are in the shrugged position, slowly roll them forward and down. Repeat this movement five to 10 times. Then do shoulder shrugs and rolls backward, and repeat this movement five to 10 times.

Biceps Stretch

Take your arms out to the sides, slightly behind your elbows, with the thumbs up. Rotate your thumbs down and back until they are pointing to the back wall. You will feel a stretch in your biceps. Repeat 3 to 5 times.

Reaching Up and Down

While sitting or standing with your arms at your sides, reach up with one hand toward the ceiling and reach down with the other hand toward the floor. Hold this stretch for 15 to 30 seconds. Repeat 3 to 5 times while alternating arms.

Anterior Shoulder Stretch

Stand in a doorway or use a sturdy object (tree, pole) with your right arm out to your side at a 90-degree angle and your elbow flexed to 90 degrees. Place your palm, forearm, and elbow on the door frame (tree/pole). Lean forward through the open door, feeling the stretch in your anterior chest and shoulder. Hold this position for 15 to 30 seconds. Repeat three to five times and then perform stretch on the opposite side.

Upper Back Stretch

Stand in an upright position, feet together with slight bend in knees. Next, clasps hands in front of body and round back towards floor, pressing arms away from body. You will feel a stretch in the upper part of your back. Keep head in a neutral (head aligned straight) position throughout movement. Hold position. Repeat three to five times.

Lower Body Stretches
(Glutes, Hamstrings and Calves)

Gluteal (buttocks) Stretch

Sit in a chair or lie on your back. Flex (bend) one knee toward your chest and place your hands around the front of your knee, pulling the knee up towards the shoulder of the same side and you will feel the stretch in your gluteal (buttocks) area. Hold position for 15 to 30 seconds. Repeat three to five times and then perform stretch on the opposite side.

Hip Flexor (hips) Stretch

Stand with your hands grasping a chair or sturdy object (tree). With your left foot supporting your body weight and right leg extended back, push your pelvis forward with your torso in the upright position, you will feel the stretch in the front of your hip. Hold this position for 15 to 30 seconds. Repeat three to five times and then perform stretch on the opposite side.

Hamstring Stretch (Standing)

While standing, place one foot forward on a bench or step with knee slightly bent. While supporting most of your weight on the other foot, lean forward at the waist with arms reaching toward your toes, you will feel the stretch in the back of your thigh (hamstrings). Hold this position for 15 to 30 seconds. Repeat three to five times and then perform stretch on the opposite side.

Hamstring Stretch (Lying Down)

Lie on your back, place one leg in the air, while opposite leg rests on the floor. With slight bend in knee, position hands underneath your knee and gently move knee towards chest, you will feel the stretch in your hamstring. Hold this position for 15 to 30 seconds. Repeat 3 to 5 times and then perform stretch on the opposite side.

Quadriceps (front part of leg) Stretch

Standing with your right hand grasping a chair for stability, hold your left ankle behind you with your left hand, pulling it upward and backward and feeling the stretch in the front of your thigh. Hold this position for 15 to 30 seconds. Repeat three to five times and then perform stretch on the opposite side.

Calf Stretch (Bent Knee)

Standing with your arms stretched in front of you and hands on a wall, support your weight on the right foot with the right knee slightly bent while placing your left foot behind you with the heel on the ground and the knee slightly bent. Lean forward, you will feel the stretch in your calf. Hold for 15 to 30 seconds. Repeat three to five times. Perform this stretch on the opposite side.

Calf Stretch (Straight Knee)

Standing with your arms stretched in front of you and hands on a wall, support your weight on your right foot with knee slightly bent while placing your left foot behind you with the heel on the ground and the knee straight. Lean forward, you will feel the stretch in your calf. Hold for 15 to 30 seconds. Repeat three to five times. Perform this stretch on the opposite side.

Chapter 28

Define Your Curves

For beginners, it is essential to slowly incorporate resistance training into your fitness training program. Therefore it is advisable to only resistance train three days per week on non-consecutive days (Monday, Wednesday, and Friday).

Doing more than three days per week at the beginning of your fitness training program may result in mental burnout and injuries. In addition to performing resistance training as a part of your new fitness training program, it is also recommended to incorporate cardiovascular exercise on the same day as your resistance training.

How does this work?

On the days in which you choose to perform both resistance training and cardiovascular activities, perform your resistance training exercises first followed by your cardiovascular activities. Later in this chapter you will find a step-by-step guide teaching you how to flow throughout your entire workout from start to finish.

Intermediate and advanced level individuals, you can incorporate resistance training five days per week for your fitness training program. At this stage, you have the strength to perform more volume. In addition to your resistance training, perform cardiovascular activities five days a week, allowing at least 48 hours of rest in between each muscle group. The body's muscle fibers are broken down when you resistance train, therefore, rest time is essential in assisting your body in recovery and repair.

Before you begin the following exercises to sculpt your curves, identify your current fitness training level. Identifying your current fitness training level will assist you in choosing the proper amount of sets, repetitions and rest time for each exercise.

Identify Your Fitness Training Level

Identify whether or not you're beginner, intermediate or advanced level. Based on your training level, determine how many sets and repetitions you will perform for each exercise.

> **Beginner:** No previous experience with resistance training or recreational activities.
>
> **Intermediate:** Train at least 3 days per week, including cardiovascular activities.
>
> **Advanced:** An athlete or you have more than a year experience with resistance training. Train at least 4-5 days per week.

Sets and Repetitions

Below you find the amount of sets and repetitions that you will perform based on your current fitness level.

> **Beginner:** Perform: 2 sets per exercise for 10-12 repetitions using light weight (5-8 lbs.). Perform modified version (MV) for each exercise that isn't within your current fitness level.
>
> **Intermediate:** Perform: 3 sets per exercise for 12-15 repetitions each using moderate weight (10-15 lbs.).
>
> **Advanced:** Perform 3-5 sets per exercise for 6-8 repetitions for strength and 12-15 repetitions for tone. Use moderate to heavier weight (15 lbs. or more).

How Does the Lifting and Training Process Work?

Use the following information to create a roadmap for the days you decide to workout. Keep in mind all of the following exercises can be done in the privacy of your own home or the gym.

If your body is not ready to incorporate the following resistance training exercises, you may stick with basic walking for 30 minutes at least five days per week until you are ready to incorporate more physical activity.

Step 1). Determine Your Days: Determine, which days of the week you are going to devote to your workouts (ex. Monday, Wednesday, and Friday). On the days that you perform your resistance training, I recommended doing at least 30 minutes are cardio. If you only have an hour to workout, split your time doing 30 minutes of resistance training and 30 minutes of cardiovascular exercise. If you only have 30 minutes for cardiovascular activities, I recommend doing intervals which consist of doing a high-level burst of activity, followed by rest for a short period of time before going back to the high-level activity (e.g. Sprint for one minute, recover by walking for 30 seconds). I will provide more examples below. On the weekends if time allows and your current fitness levels allows, complete at least 45 minutes of cardiovascular activities.

Step 2). Determine Which Body Part(s): Once you have determined which days of the week you're going to train, determine which muscle(s) you're going to train. Below you have been given exercises that are grouped by two muscle groups. The way the groups were created was to try both a primary and secondary muscle group (e.g. Bicep and Triceps). You can choose to do both muscle groups or you can choose to only do one group. I'd prefer you train the way I have designed the program to get the most effective and efficient workout.

Step 3). Warm-Up Properly: Before each workout session perform a warm-up for at least five to 10 minutes. The warm-up is essential in increasing your core temperature and prepares your body for your workout. NEVER skip a warm-up. Doing so can increase your risk of injury which can lead to chronic issues if left untreated.

Step 4). Have your plan ready: Before arriving at the gym, know which muscle groups you're going to train. Once you have completed your warm-up go straight to performing your resistance training exercises. Stay focused and move from one exercise to another in a circuit fashion if your current fitness level allows you to accomplish this. Don't rest any longer than 30 seconds after one set of exercises or no longer than 90 seconds after a complete circuit.

Step 5). Cardio Time: Once you have completed your resistance training routine, go straight to your cardiovascular program. By this time your core temperature in raised and you can go straight into your activity of choice.

Step 6: Stretch Please: Once you have completed your cardio, if time allows, stretch each large muscle group in what is known as a static hold stretch for 15 to 30 seconds. At all times only stretch as far as your body naturally will allow you to. Do not bounce while you're stretching and do not stretch cold muscles! Perform at least one to two stretches per large muscle group.

Nutrition Guidelines:

- ✓ For optimal performance ensure you are eating at least two hours before your training session. If you're training at a high intensity beyond one hour, it may be essential to replenish your glycogen (sugar) stores with an intra-workout drink such Gatorade or PowerAde. Drink only when needed due to the amount of sugar found in these drinks.

- ✓ Consume a healthy source of protein and carbohydrates before your workouts. Carbohydrates are your bodies' main fuel source and when consumed with a healthy source of protein, can sustain your energy levels throughout your workouts. (E.g. A peanut butter and banana sandwich, protein drink and one piece of fruit).
- ✓ Drink water before, during and after each workout. Water assists your body in temperature regulation during workouts.

Technique Guidelines:
- ✓ At all times maintain proper form and never jeopardize form to make increases in the amount of weight you desire to lift. The key to progress is to perform EACH movement with proper form with an amount of weight that is appropriate to your current fitness level.
- ✓ Allow at least 24to 48 hours between each training session of each muscle group to avoid overtraining and to recover properly. You may experience soreness which may peak 24 to 48 hours after your training session. This is referred to as Delayed Onset Muscle Soreness or DOMS. This is a natural effect of exercise however, listen to your bodies signals. If you remain sore for longer than 72 hours you may need to drop your amount of weight, sets and repetitions.

Tighten, Firm and Tone

A toned upper body not only looks great for the warmer months when sleeveless shirts and swimsuits are worn, but toned arms are also great for assisting you in activities of daily living such as picking up your children, carrying groceries, and being able to lift and carry your laundry. Research has shown that after the age of 30 women begin to lose muscle tissue by three to five percent per decade. A loss of muscle tissue can lead to diminished mobility and strength in the aging process. Therefore, it is essential to incorporate resistance training into your normal fitness regimen on a regular basis.

The following exercises in this chapter will help you sculpt and tone your upper body without adding a bulky appearance. Discover your skill level and perform the exercises prescribed to you. If you are a beginner, listen to your body and only perform the amount of sets and repetitions that feel appropriate for you. Intermediate and advanced levels - don't be afraid to safely push your body by adding extra resistance and increasing your repetitions.

Chest Exercises

Movement Tip: To avoid injury, keep core contracted throughout entire movement. Doing so will keep body aligned and lessen the chance of injury to your back.

Beginner Level

Exercise	Sets	Repetitions
One-Arm Med Ball Pushups *Modified Version	2-3	4-6
Single-Legged Chest Press	2-3	8-10 each arm
Physio-ball Chest Press	2-3	10-12 each arm
Resistance Band Flyes	2-3	10-12

Intermediate Level

Exercise	Sets	Repetitions
One-Arm Med Ball Pushups	3-4	15-20
Single-Legged Chest Press	3-4	15-20 each arm
Physio-ball Chest Press	3-4	15-20 each arm
Physio-ball Pushups	3-4	10-15
Resistance Band Flyes	3-4	12-15

Advanced Level

Exercise	Sets	Repetitions
One-Arm Med Ball Pushups	4-5	15
Single-Legged Chest Press	4-5	15
Physio-ball Chest Press	4-5	15 each arm
One-Arm Med Ball Pushups	4-5	15
Resistance Band Flyes	4-5	15-20

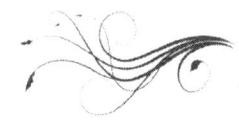

Upper Body Exercises

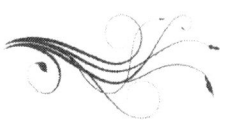

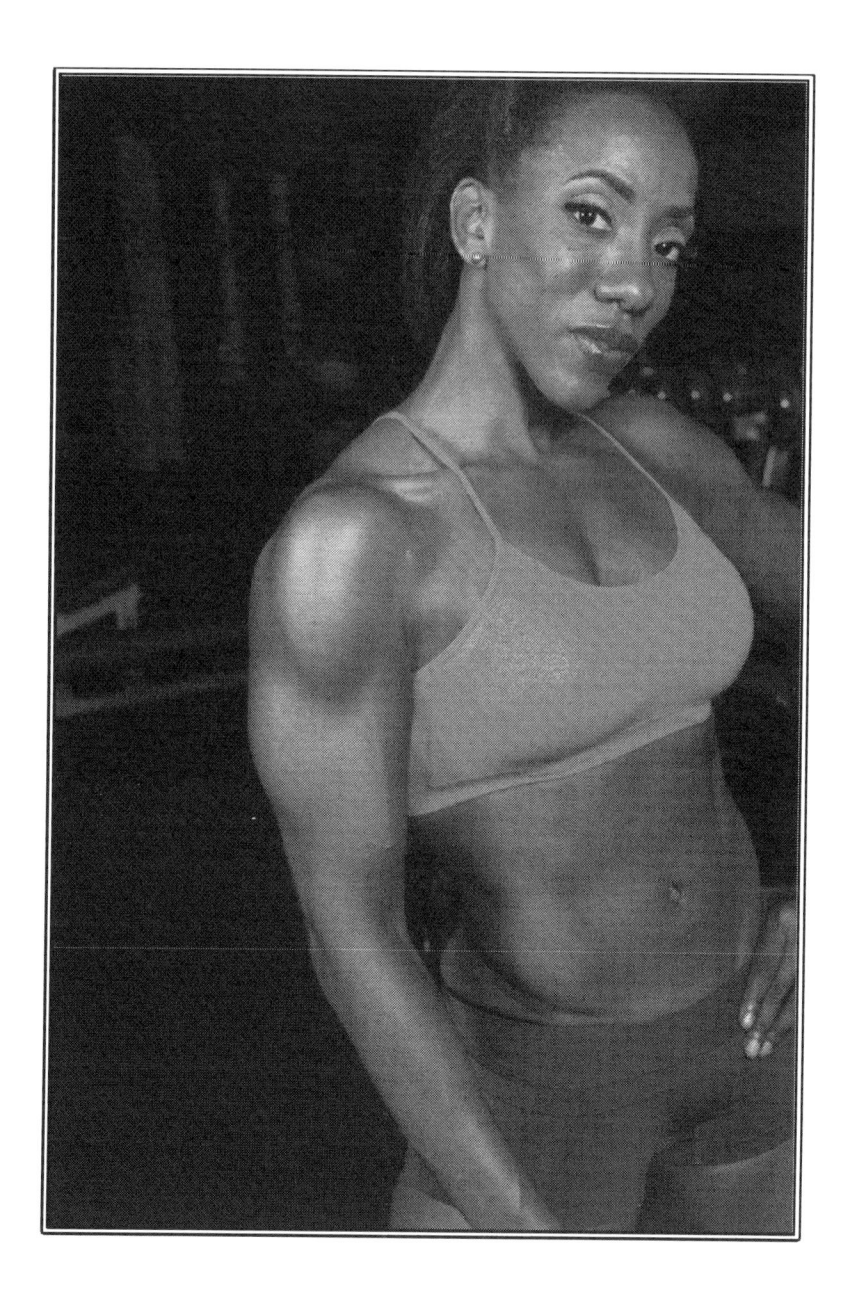

CHANGING THE NORM

One-Arm Med Ball Pushups

Targeted Muscles: chest, triceps

Set Up: Kneel on the ground with hands positioned shoulder width apart, one hand resting on med ball with other hand placed on ground. From kneeling position, extend arms and legs.

Action: In a slow and controlled manner, bend your elbows and lower your body until arms form a 90-degree angle. Hold for a count and then extend your arms and push body back to starting position. Complete set and then switch arms.

Movement Tip: To avoid back injury, keep core tight and body in straight position. Do not drop hips.

*****Modified Version:** Perform exercise on your knees.

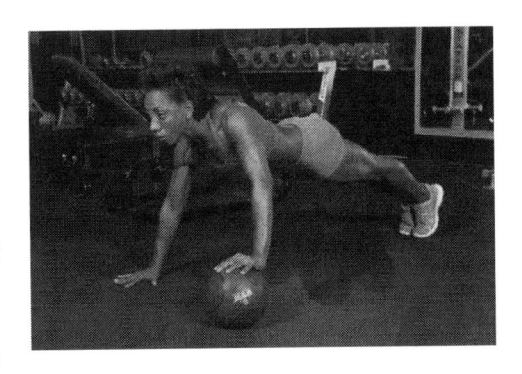

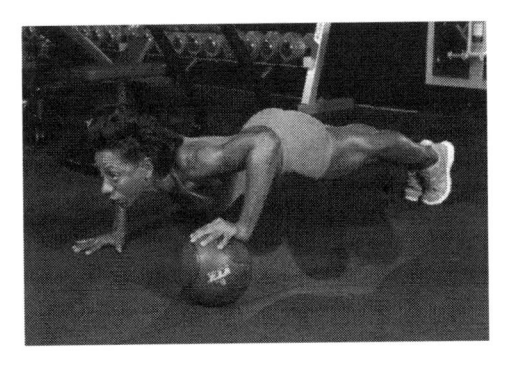

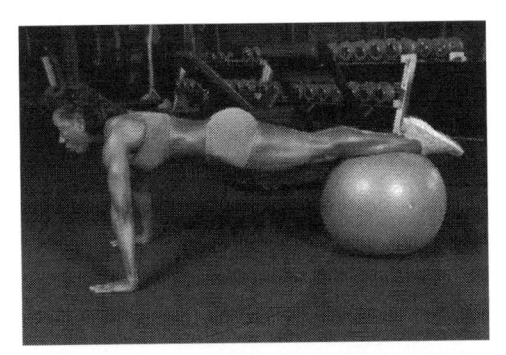

Physio-ball Pushups

Targeted Muscles: chest, triceps

Set Up: Place stability ball in front of body. Slowly roll your body onto the ball until your shins rest on ball. Your arms are positioned shoulder width apart with lower body and core tight. Keep slight bend in elbows.

Action: In a slow and controlled manner, bend elbows and slowly lower body until your arms form a 90- degree angle. Hold for a count and then extend arms to return body to starting position. Repeat movement until set is complete.

Movement Tip: To avoid injury, keep core tight throughout entire movement.

Single-Legged Chest Press

Targeted Muscles: glutes, hamstrings, chest, triceps

Set Up: Lay on back with both feet on ground, knees bent with arms bent holding dumbbells at chest level.

Action: In an upward movement, slowly bridge up on one leg, with opposite leg elevated off ground. Once lower body is off ground, press dumbbell upward until arms are fully extended. Hold for a count and then bring body back to starting position. Complete set and then switch to opposite arm and leg.

*Modified Version: Keep both feet on ground. Maintain body in bridged position.

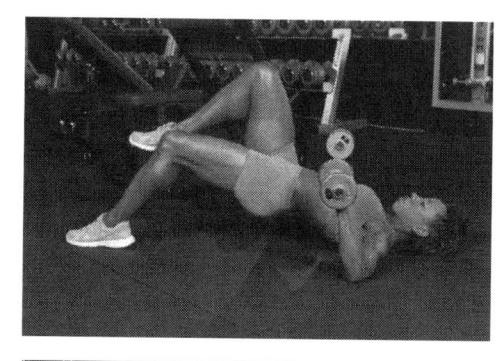

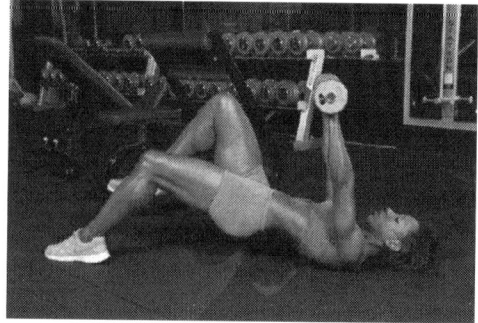

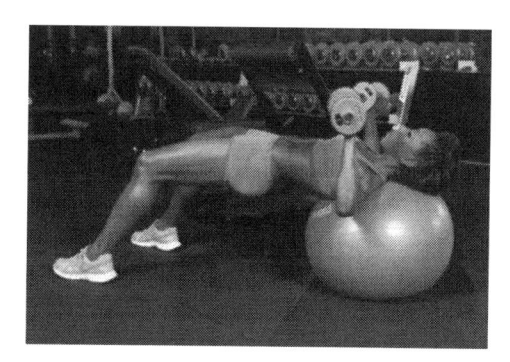

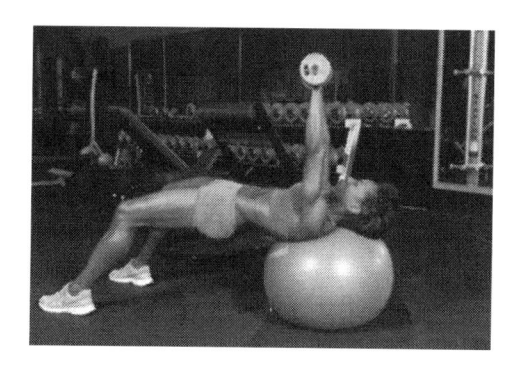

Physio-ball Chest Press

Targeted Muscles: chest, triceps

Set Up: Position body on a stability ball with a pair of dumbbells in both hands with feet positioned apart. In a slow and controlled manner, slowly walk your feet away from the ball until your upper back rests on stability ball. Elbows are bent with dumbbells facing inward with hips parallel to floor and feet positioned slightly apart.

Action: In a slow and controlled manner, slowly lower weight to sides of upper chest until slight stretch is felt in chest or shoulder. Hold for a count and then slowly extend arms to starting position without locking elbows. Keep core engaged and hips elevated in order to maintain form throughout entire movement.

Movement Tip: Keep hips and core contracted.

*Modified Version: Drop hips to mid-level. Keep core contracted at all times.

Around the World

Targeted Muscles: chest, triceps
Set Up: Begin in pushup position with hands shoulder width apart, body in a straight line, core and lower body tight.

Action: In a slow and controlled manner, slowly bend your elbows and lower body until you reach a 90-degree angle. Hold for a count and then extend your arms and return to starting position. While in starting pushup position, lift right arm and rotate arm across body and hold for a count. Bring arm down. Perform another pushup and then repeat lift with opposite arm.

*Modified Version: Perform exercise on knees.

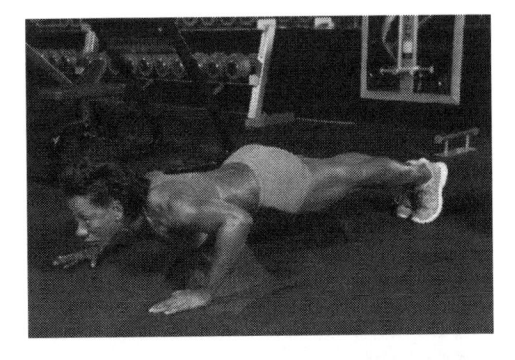

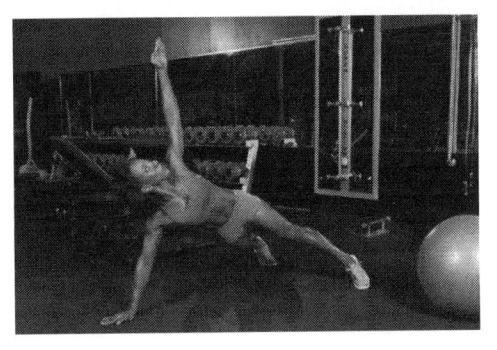

Fit Tip: This Is An Advanced Movement Therefore Only Try If You've Exercised Your Core On A Regular Basis.

CHANGING THE NORM

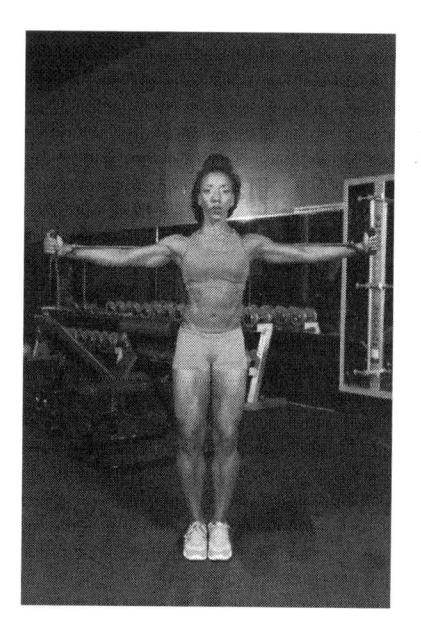

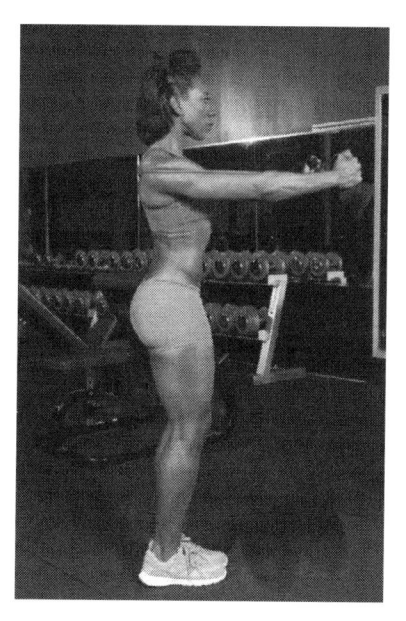

Resistance Bands Flyes

Targeted Muscles: chest, triceps

Set Up: While in a standing position, with chest up shoulder blades back and slight bend in knees, grab resistant band and place behind the back of your shoulders. Once band is placed behind shoulders place a bend in elbows with arms extended out to the side of your body.

Action: With a slight bend in elbows, squeeze chest muscles together and bring arms together with palms facing one another. Hold for account and bring arms back to starting position. Repeat until set is complete.

FIT TIP:

Using resistance training bands is a non-expensive and fun way to get fit at the gym, at home or while you travel.

If you travel often, packing a resistance training band in your suitcase will allow you to stay fit on the go. You can get fit and creative with resistance training bands!

Back Exercise

Movement Tip: Keep core contracted while performing each exercise. This will keep body aligned and lessen the chance of injury to your back.

Beginner Level

Exercise	Sets	Repetitions
Seated Resistance Band Rows	2-3	10-12
One-Arm Row	2-3	10-12
Two-Arm Row *Modified Version	2-3	10-12

Intermediate Level

Exercise	Sets	Repetitions
Seated Resistance Band Rows	3-4	15-20
One-Arm Row	3-4	15-20
Two-Arm Row	3-4	15-20

Advanced Level

Exercise	Sets	Repetitions
Seated Resistance Band Rows	4-5	8-15
One-Arm Row	4-5	8-15
Two-Arm Row	4-5	15

Seated Resistance Band Rows

Targeted Muscles: back, chest
Set Up: While in a seated position, shoulder back, core engaged and chest up, with knees bent and heels on the ground, place resistance band under the base of your shoe, grasping both handles with arms fully extended.

Action: In a slow and controlled manner, bring elbows back by squeezing shoulder blades together. Hold for a count and repeat entire movement until set is complete.

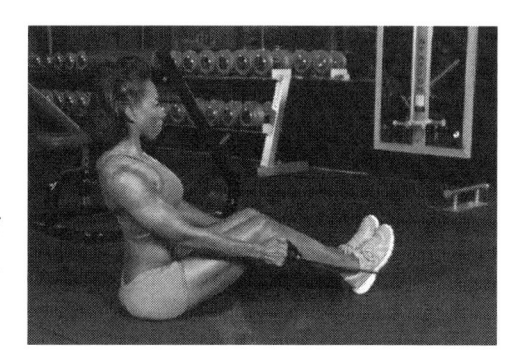

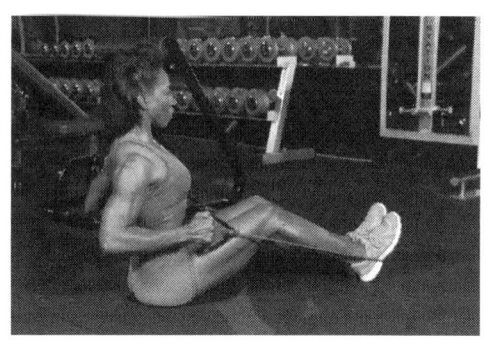

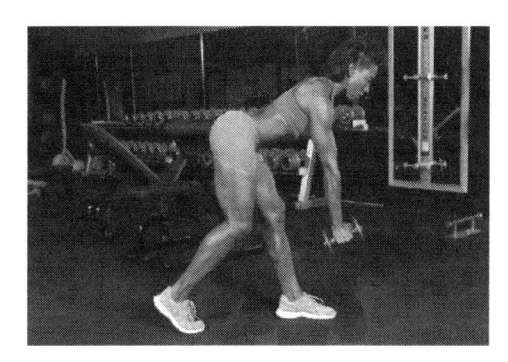

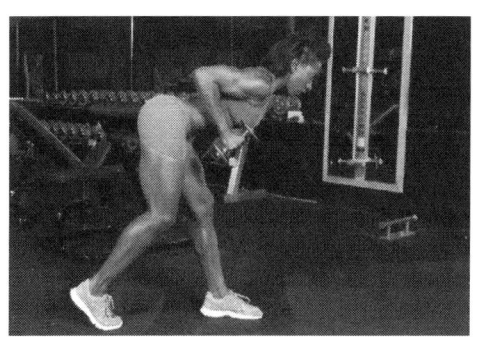

One-Arm Row

Targeted Muscles: back, core
Set Up: Begin by standing in a split stance, with one foot staggered in front of the other. Place a slight bend in knees, arm holding dumbbells in front of body with slight lean in torso.

Action: In a slow and controlled manner with core engaged, bring elbow back by squeezing your shoulder blade. Hold for a count and then extend arm back to starting position. Complete movement until set is complete and then switch arms.

Two-Arm Row

Targeted Muscles: back, core

Set Up: Begin by standing in a split stance, with one foot staggered in front of the other. Place a slight bend in knees, lean in torso, with arms extended in front of body holding dumbbells.

Action: In a slow and controlled manner with core engaged, bring elbows back by squeezing your shoulder blades together. Hold for a count and then extend arms back to starting position. Complete movement until set is complete.

*Modified Version: Keep torso forward, but keep back leg on the ground.

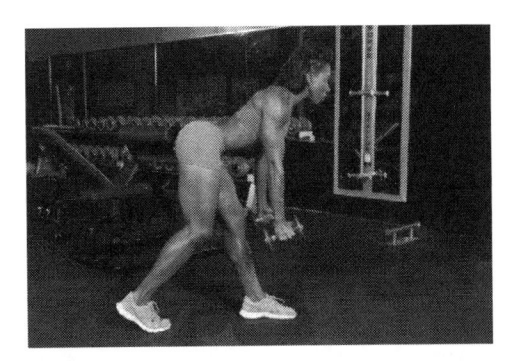

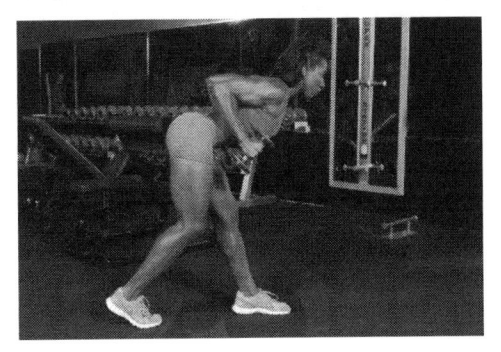

Movement Tip:

Keep Your Eyes and Head Straight!

Shoulder Exercises

Movement Tip: Keep core contracted while performing each exercise. This will keep body aligned and lessen the chance of injury to your back.

Beginner Level

Exercise	Sets	Repetitions
Core Shoulder Lifts *Modified Version	2-3	8-10
Front Shoulder Raises	2-3	10-12
Lateral Shoulder Raises	2-3	10-12
Rear Shoulder Raises	2-3	10-12

Intermediate Level

Exercise	Sets	Repetitions
Core Shoulder Lifts	3-4	10-12
Front Shoulder Raises	3-4	15-20
Lateral Shoulder Raises	3-4	15-20
Rear Shoulder Raises	3-4	15-20

Advanced Level

Exercise	Sets	Repetitions
Core Shoulder Lifts*	4	12-15
Front Shoulder Raises	4-5	8-15
Lateral Shoulder Raises	4-5	8-15
Rear Shoulder Raises	4-5	8-15

*Use a heavier medicine ball around 8-10 lbs. for added resistance

Core Shoulder Lifts

Targeted Muscles: anterior deltoids (front shoulder), core

Set Up: Position body on a mat with feet flat on floor, knees bent, chest up and arms extended in front of body while holding medicine ball.

Action: With core tight, in a slow and controlled manner, slightly lean back and raise feet about two inches off ground (Advanced level can raise feet higher). Once stabilized in position, lift arms in an upward position. Hold for a count, and then bring arms down. Repeat movement.

Movement Tip: Keep core tight and chest up to avoid rounding back while performing movement.

*Modified Version: Keep both feet on ground.

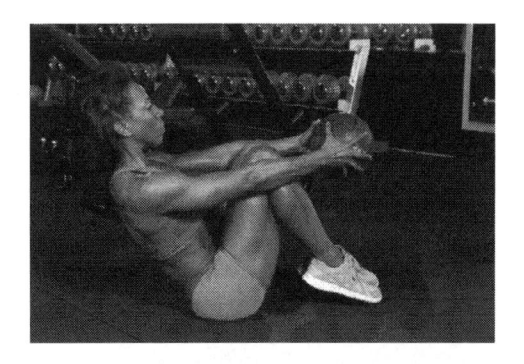

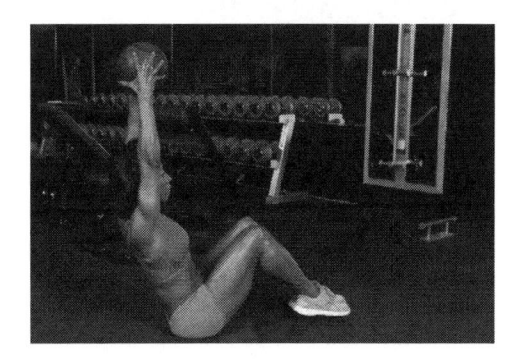

FIT JEWEL: HAVING A STRONG CORE HELPS YOU PERFORM ALL OF YOUR DAY TO DAY TASKS WITH BETTER EASE!

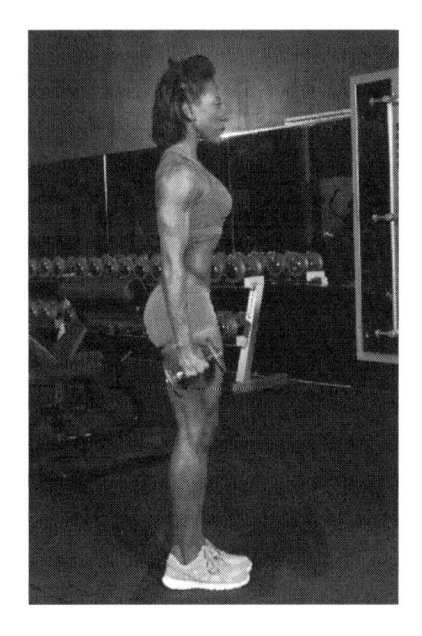

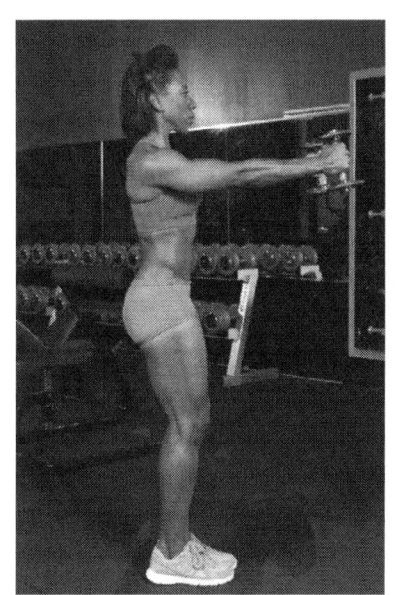

Front Shoulder Raises

Targeted Muscles: anterior deltoids (front shoulder)

Set up: Stand in an upright position, feet positioned together or apart, core engaged with slight bend in knees. Dumbbells held in a neutral (palms facing inward towards your body) position in your hands.

Action: In a slow and controlled manner lift dumbbells in an upward movement raising arms until they reach eye level with palms facing each other. Hold for a count and then return hands back to starting position.

Movement tip: Keep slight bend in knees throughout the entire movement and don't allow body to swing as you move the dumbbells away from your body. Keep core engaged and feet anchored to ground in order to avoid swinging movement.

FIT JEWEL

Hello summer and short sleeve shirts!

Lateral Shoulder Raises

Targeted Muscles: lateral deltoids (middle of shoulder)

Set Up: Stand with your feet together, knees slightly bent, while holding dumbbells facing inward towards your hips.

Action: With a slight bend in elbows, in a slow and controlled manner, lift arms in a lateral position (lateral means away from the mid-line of your body) until arms are parallel to the floor. Hold for a count and then lower arms back to starting position. Repeat movement until set is complete.

Movement Tip: Do not bring arms too high. As a reference point, you should be able to see the back of your hands in your peripheral view. If you can't see your hands, you're lifting too high. Raising arms to high releases tension off shoulder and places stress on other muscles. Do not arch back throughout movement.

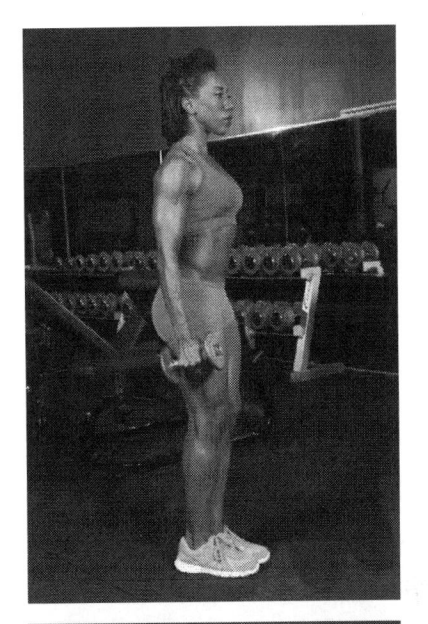

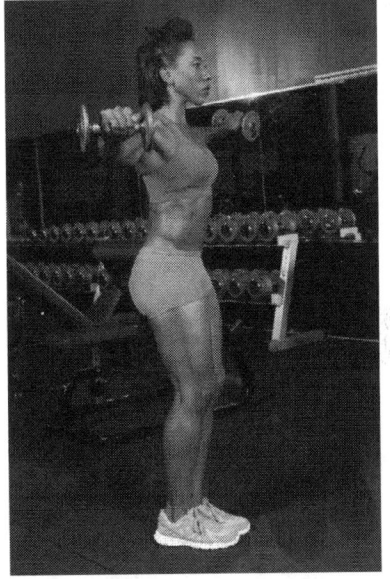

FIT JEWEL

Toned shoulders look great regardless of what you wear, therefore don't forget to incorporate shoulder exercises into your fitness training program.

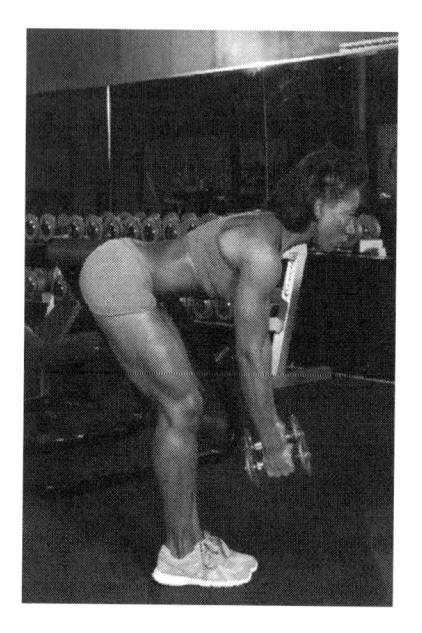

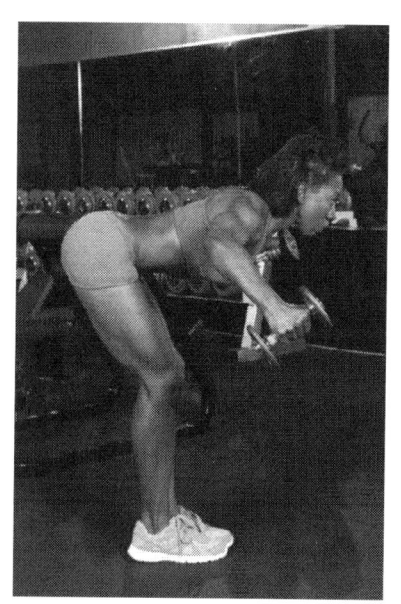

Rear Shoulder Raises

Targeted Muscles: rear deltoids, core

Set Up: Begin with feet together, knees bent, torso forward with arms extended in front of body holding dumbbells facing inward towards body.

Action: With a slight bend in elbows, in a slow and controlled manner, lift arms away from body in an arching movement by squeezing shoulder blades together. Hold for a count and then lower arms back to starting position. Repeat movement until set is complete.

Movement Tip: Keep knees bent and core tight.

FIT JEWEL

Nice toned shoulders are great for the winter, summer or anytime of the year!

Biceps Exercises

Movement Tip: Keep core contracted while performing each exercise. This will keep body aligned and lessen the chance of injury to your back.

Beginner Level

Exercise	Sets	Repetitions
Kneeling Physio-ball Curls	2-3	8-10
Single-Legged Bicep Curls *Modified Version	2-3	8-10
Split Stance Hammer Curls	2-3	8-10
Resistance Bands Curls	2-3	8-10

Intermediate Level

Exercise	Sets	Repetitions
Kneeling Physio-ball Curls	3-4	10-12
Single-Legged Bicep Curls	3-4	10-12
Split Stance Bicep Curls	3-4	10-12
Resistance Bands Curls	3-4	10-12

Advanced Level

Exercise	Sets	Repetitions
Kneeling Physio-ball Curls	4-5	12-15
Single-Legged Bicep Curls	4-5	12-15
Split Stance Bicep Curls	4-5	12-15
Resistance Bands Curls	4-5	12-15

Core Shoulder Lifts

Targeted Muscles: anterior deltoids (front shoulder), core

Set Up: Position body on a mat with feet flat on floor, knees bent, chest up and arms extended in front of body while holding medicine ball.

Action: With core tight, in a slow and controlled manner, slightly lean back and raise feet about two inches off ground (Advanced level can raise feet higher). Once stabilized in position, lift arms in an upward position. Hold for a count, and then bring arms down. Repeat movement.

Movement Tip: Keep core tight and chest up to avoid rounding back while performing movement.

***Modified Version**: Keep both feet on ground.

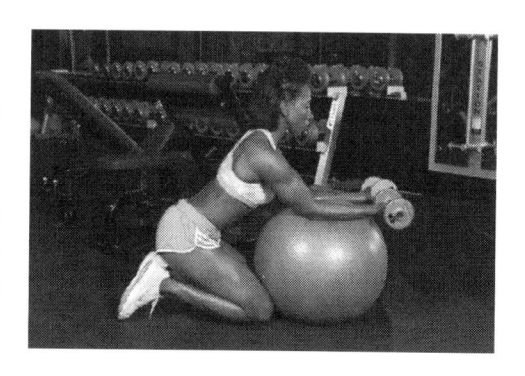

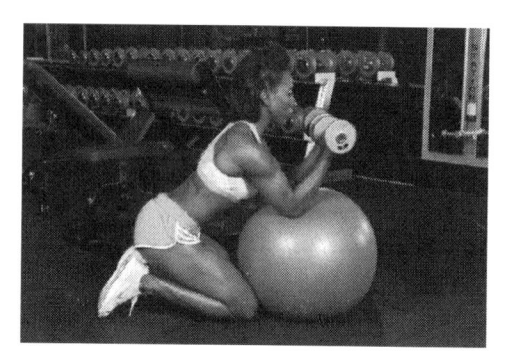

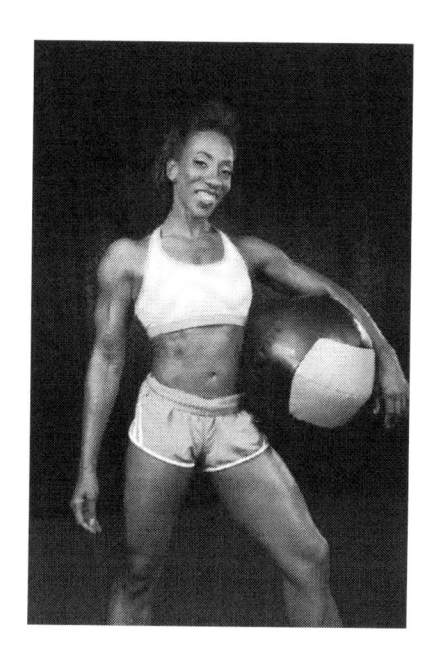

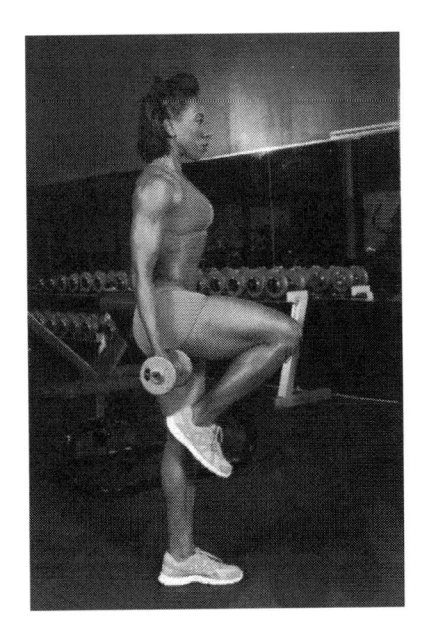

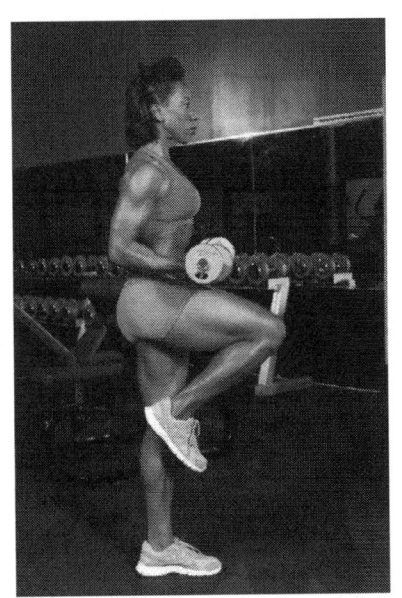

Rear Shoulder Raises

Targeted Muscles: rear deltoids, core

Set Up: Begin with feet together, knees bent, torso forward with arms extended in front of body holding dumbbells facing inward towards body.

Action: With a slight bend in elbows, in a slow and controlled manner, lift arms away from body in an arching movement by squeezing shoulder blades together. Hold for a count and then lower arms back to starting position. Repeat movement until set is complete.

Movement Tip: Keep knees bent and core tight.

FIT JEWEL

While standing on one leg, keep core engaged this will help you keep your balance.

Split Stance Hammer Curls

Targeted Muscles: biceps

Set Up: In an upright position stagger feet evenly positioning body weight on front and back legs, with shoulders back, core engaged while holding dumbbells in a neutral position (palms facing towards your body), with slight bend in elbows.

Action: In a slow and controlled manner, slowly squeeze biceps and bring dumbbells towards your shoulder while keeping elbows positioned close to your body. Hold for a count and then return hands to starting position without fully extending arms. Repeat movement until set is complete.

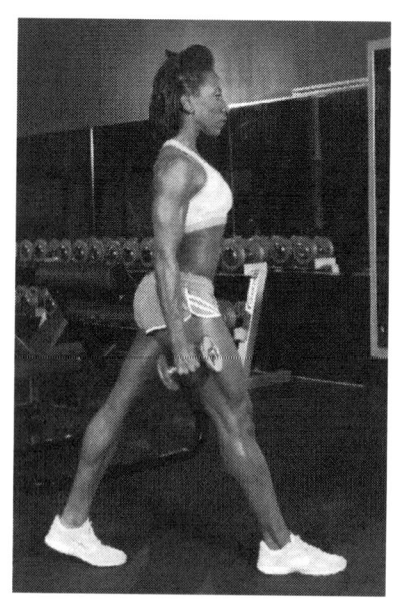

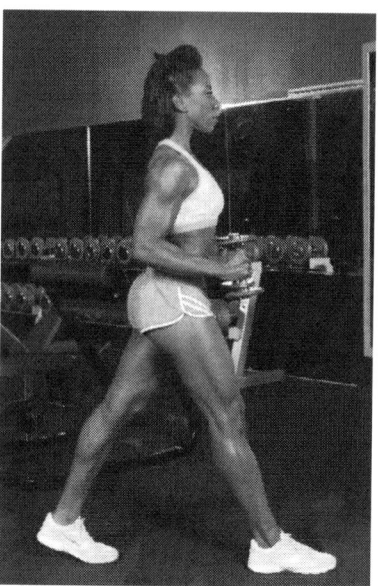

FIT JEWEL

Never jeopardize form for weight. If you can't properly lift the weight you're using, decrease the amount of weight.

CHANGING THE NORM

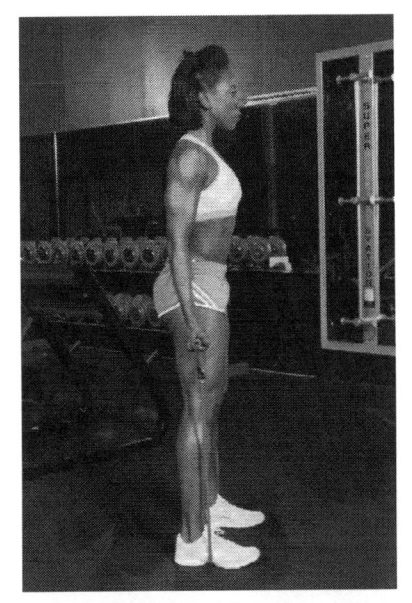

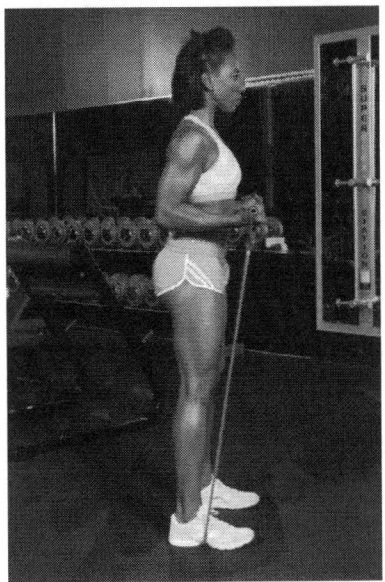

Resistance Bands Curls

Targeted Muscles: biceps

Set Up: Place resistance band underneath both feet creating enough space to create equal resistance on handles. Once band is placed under feet, stand in an upright position with shoulders back, core engaged, slight bend in knees and palms facing upward with resistance band in both hands.

Action: In a slow and controlled manner with elbows close to body, squeeze biceps and bring hands towards shoulders, hold for a count and then return hands to starting position without fully extending arms.

Movement Tip: Keep a slight bend in knees at all times in order to avoid placing stress on your lower back. When performing movement, do not allow elbows to move away from the body, doing so will place less stress on biceps.

FIT JEWEL

Keep elbows locked into your side in order to fully make the biceps work.

Triceps Exercises

Movement Tip: Keep core contracted while performing each exercise. This will keep body aligned and lessen the chance of injury to your back.

Beginner Level

Exercise	Sets	Repetitions
Resistance Band Extensions	1-2	8-10
Standing Triceps Kickbacks	1-2	8-10
Seated Overhead Triceps Extensions *Modified Version	1-2	8-10

Intermediate Level

Exercise	Sets	Repetitions
Resistance Band Extensions	2-3	10-12
Standing Triceps Kickbacks	2-3	10-12
Seated Overhead Triceps Extensions	2-3	10-12
Pyramid Pushups	2-3	10-12

Advanced Level

Exercise	Sets	Repetitions
Resistance Band Extensions	3-4	12-15
Standing Triceps Kickbacks	3-4	12-15
Seated Overhead Triceps Extensions	3-4	12-15
Physio-ball Triceps Pushups	3-4	12-15

Resistance Band Extensions

Targeted Muscles: Triceps

Set Up: Place resistance band underneath the back of your foot and then stand in an upright position staggering feet evenly in order to position body weight on front and back legs. Shoulders back, core engaged while holding resistance band in hand with elbow bent.

Action: In a slow and controlled manner, contract core and fully extend arm by squeezing triceps without locking out your elbow. Hold for a count and then return arm back to starting position. Repeat movement until set is complete and then switch your arm and foot.

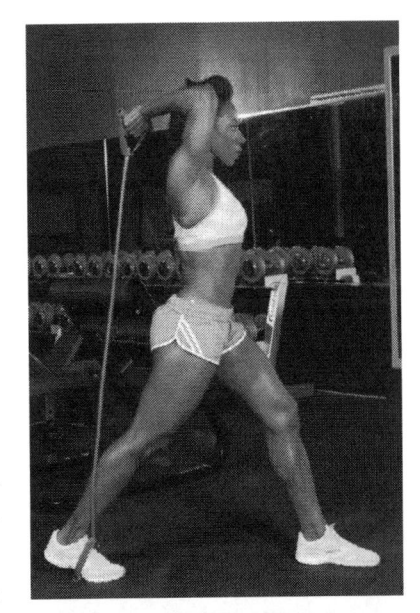

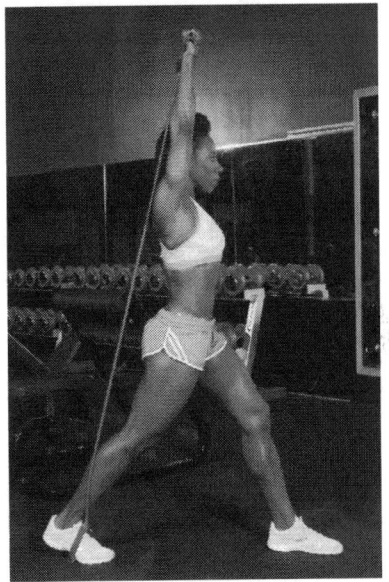

FIT JEWEL

Performing these exercises will give you the confidence to wave goodbye!

One-Arm Triceps Extensions

Targeted Muscles: triceps, core

Set Up: Place body in push up position, with hands positioned shoulder width apart. Legs spread apart to form a V with dumbbells in front of body.

Action: While contracting core, slowly grab dumbbell off floor and lift right arm off ground, tucking right elbow at side. Once elbow is tucked into side, in a slow and controlled manner, extend arm without locking out. Repeat movement until set is complete and then switch arms. Complete set with opposite arm.

Movement Tip: To avoid back injuries, keep core contracted throughout entire movement.

*Modified version: Perform on knees.

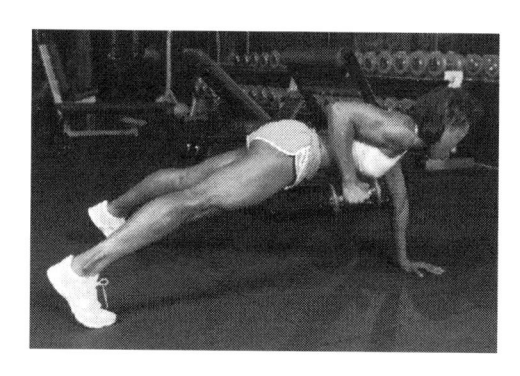

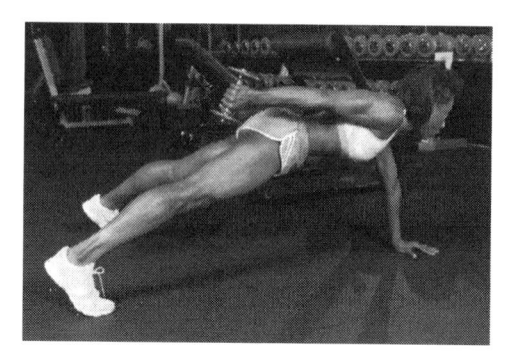

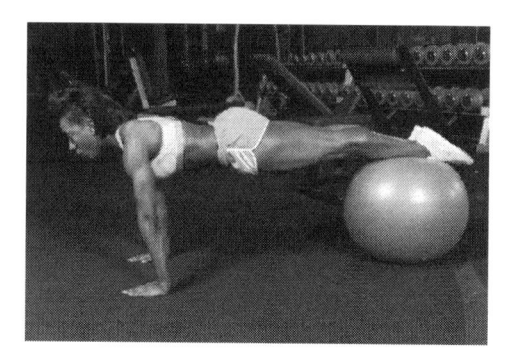

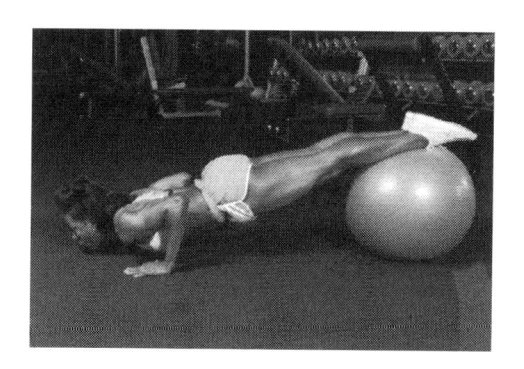

Physio-ball Triceps Pushups

Targeted Muscles: triceps, core

Set Up: In a slow and controlled manner, roll body forward onto stability ball until shins are resting on ball. Hands are positioned closer than shoulder width, with slight bend in elbows.

Action: In a slow and controlled manner, bend elbows in a hinge movement and lower body about 2-4 inches from the ground. Hold for a count and then extend arms to return body to starting position. Repeat movement until set is complete.

Movement Tip: To help balance on ball, keep core contracted and lower body aligned.

*Modified Version: Do not use ball, instead use mat and perform exercise on knees. Keep core tight throughout entire movement.

CHANGING THE NORM

Standing Triceps Kickbacks

Targeted Muscles: triceps, core

Set Up : Stand with feet together, slight bend in knees. Torso forward and elbows tucked into side of body while holding dumbbells in a supinated position (hands facing upwards towards your body).

Action: In a slow and controlled manner, extend your arms by squeezing your triceps. Hold for a count and then bring arms back to starting position. Repeat movement until set is complete.

Movement Tip: Fully extend arms without locking elbows.

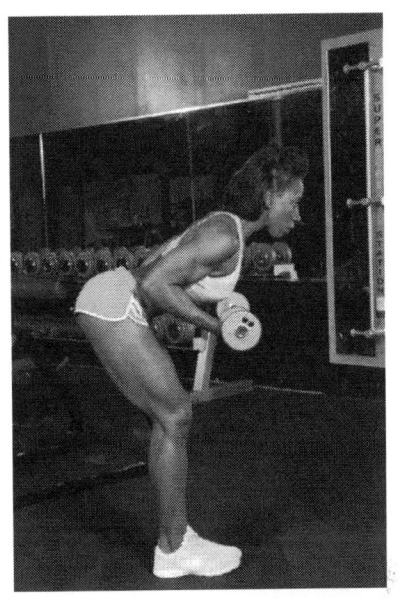

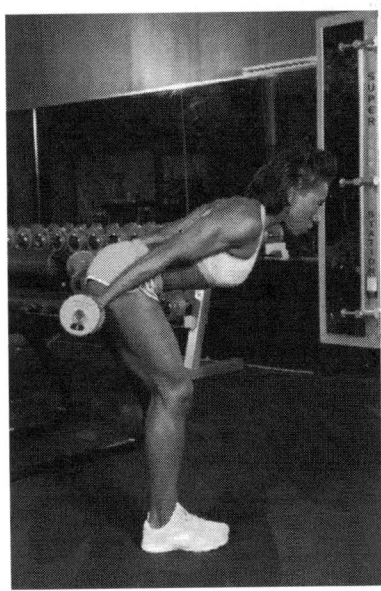

Fit Jewel

To avoid overuse injuries at the elbow joint, don't lock out elbows on triceps exercises.

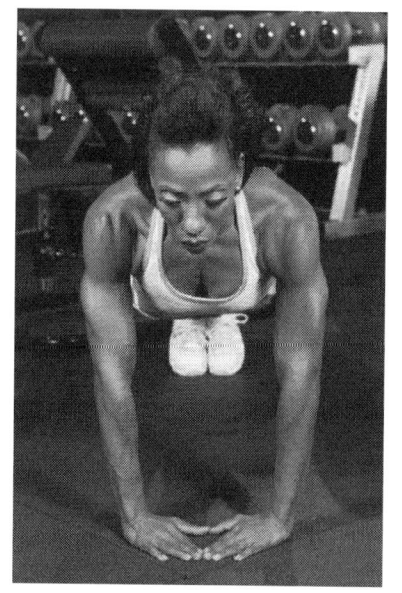

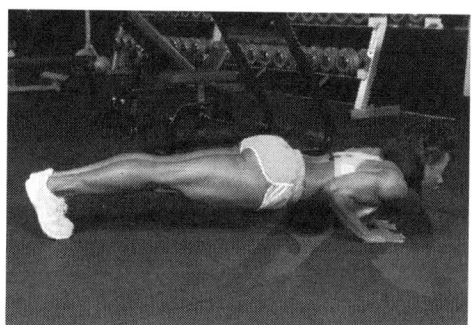

Pyramid Pushups

Targeted Muscles: triceps, core and chest

Set Up: Start with body in a pushup position, hands are positioned close together with index fingers and thumbs touching to form a diamond. Lower body and core remain aligned and contracted.

Action: In a slow and controlled manner, bend elbows and lower body parallel to floor. Once arms are positioned at 90-degrees, stop movement. Hold for a count and then extend arms to return to starting position. Repeat movement until set is complete. Do not lockout elbows when returning to starting position.

Movement Tip: To avoid back injuries, keep core tight throughout entire movement.

***Modified Version**: Perform exercise on knees.

FIT JEWEL

Many women have weaker upper bodies, but performing this exercise will help improve your upper body strength and tone your arms.

Seated Overhead Triceps Extensions

Targeted Muscles: triceps, core

Set Up: Place body on a stability ball while holding dumbbells. In a slow and controlled manner, walk your feet away from ball until your upper back rests on stability ball. Hips parallel to the floor with arms extended holding dumbbells.

Action: While maintaining balance on stability ball, in a slow and controlled manner, bend elbows and lower weight until your elbows are fully bent. Hold for a count and then extend arms back to starting position. Repeat movement until set is complete.

*****Movement Tip**: Extend arms without locking elbows.

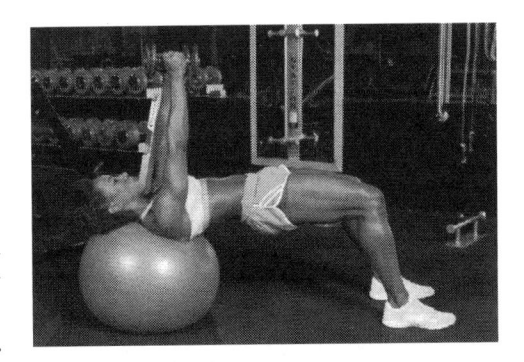

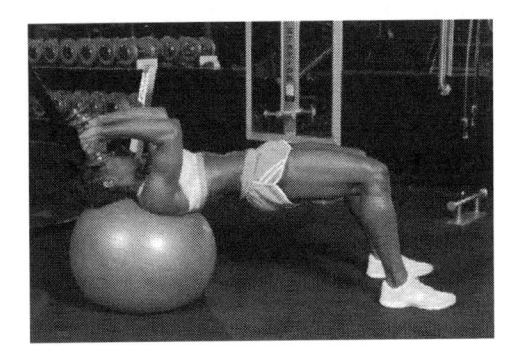

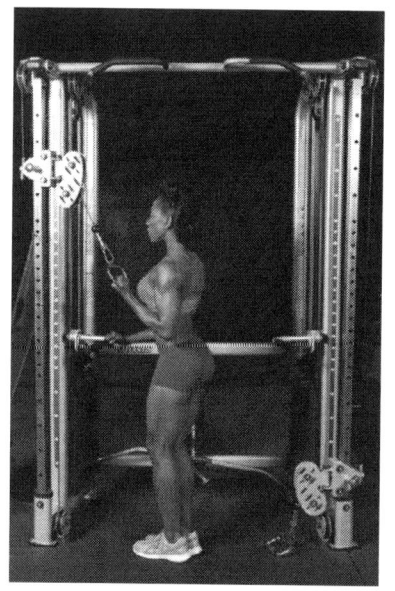

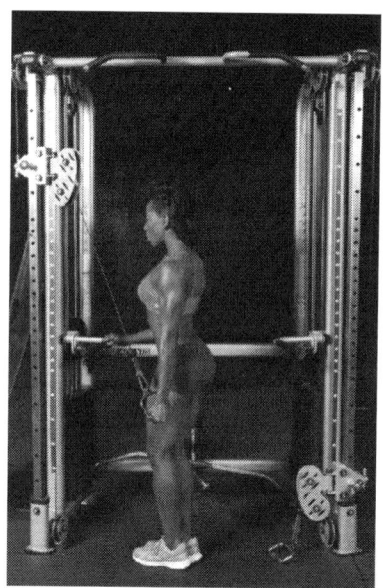

Straight Arm Extensions

Targeted Muscles: triceps, core

Set up: Stand in an upright position with body facing towards triceps extension attachment either on a Smith Machine or Universal Cable System. Shoulder blades back, slight bend in knees, core engaged and hand positioned in supinated position (palms facing upward).

Action: In a slow and controlled manner fully extend arm by squeezing triceps. Extend arm without locking elbow. Hold for a count and then return arm back to starting position. Repeat movement until set is complete and then switch arms.

FIT JEWEL

Using the cable machine is a great way to add variety into your resistance training program.

Physio-ball Overhead Triceps Extensions

Targeted Muscles: triceps, core

Set Up: Sit on physio-ball with slight bend in knees, feet flat on ground, core engaged, shoulders back and arms extended holding dumbbells.

Action: While maintaining stability on ball, in a slow and controlled manner, bend elbows and lower weight until your hands are behind your head. Hold for a count and then extend arms back to starting position. Repeat movement until set is complete.

Movement Tip: Extend arms without locking elbows out.

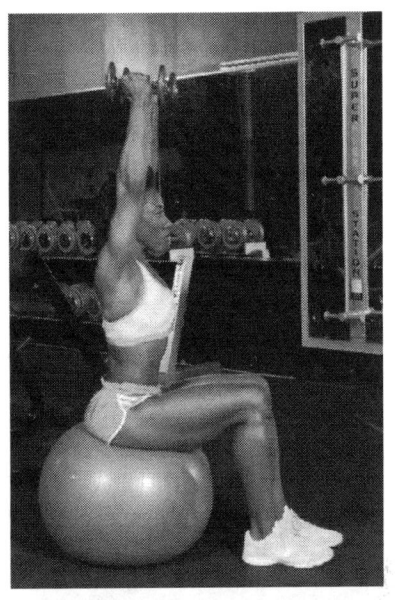

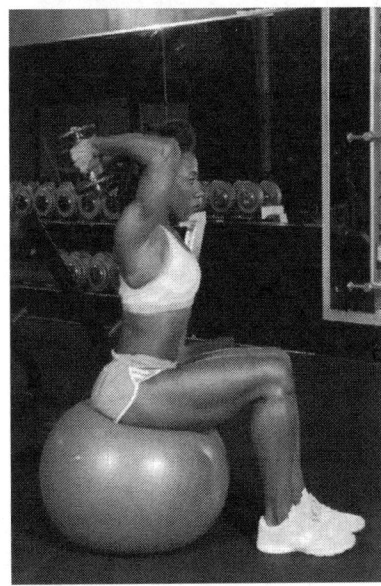

FIT JEWEL

Performing exercises on an unstable object such as the physio-ball is a great way to build core strength and balance.

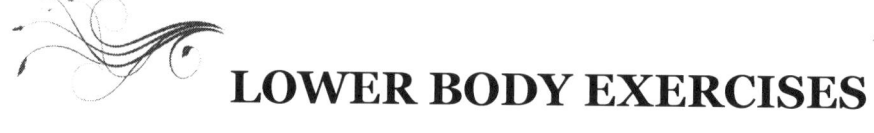

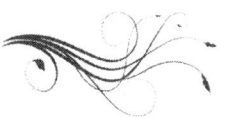

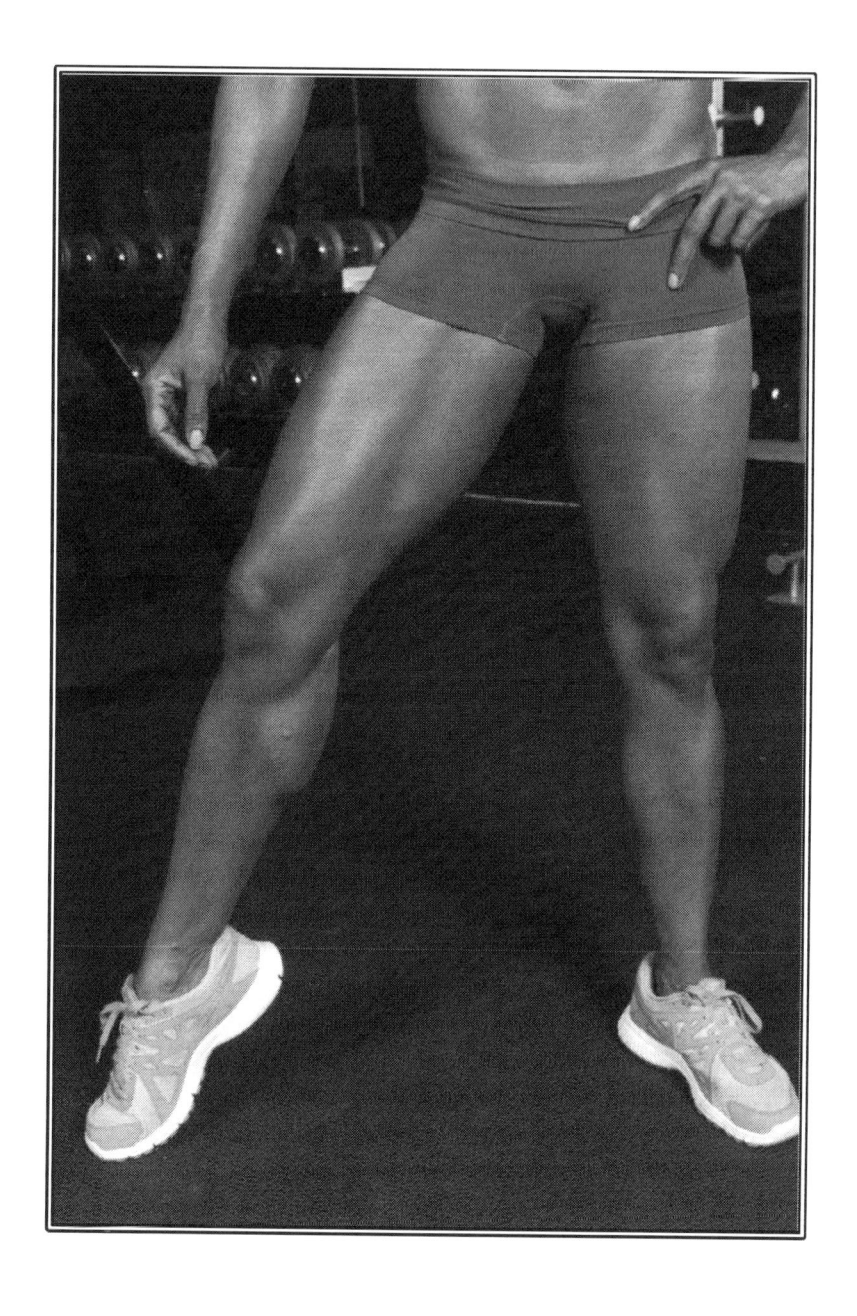

LOWER BODY EXERCISES

CHANGING THE NORM

Hips, Glutes and Thighs, Oh My!

Have you ever turned around and looked at your backside and thought, "I wish my backside was firmer?" Whether you are 26 or 46, at some point in time most women have made this statement to themselves. The backside, or the glutes and the thighs, for many women are the hardest and most challenging area to firm, tighten and tone. Women naturally carry more body fat in these areas, and as a result find it harder to see the tone they desire. Do you find it hard to tone these areas of your body?

If this is you, the exercises on the following pages are designed not only to help you look great in your favorite jeans, but the following exercises are also designed to help you keep your legs strong enough to run, bike, dance and perform all other activities of living. A firmer backside and toned legs are only a few squats away, what are you waiting for?

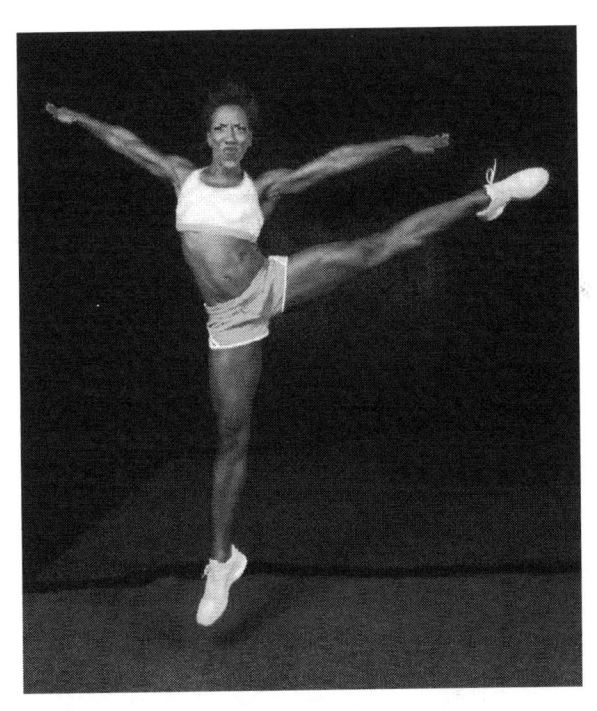

Toned legs not only look great in a pair of jeans or shorts, they are also great for jumping, picking up your kids and other sporting activities and life activities!

Lower Body Exercises

Movement Tip: Keep core contracted while performing each exercise. This will keep body aligned and lessen the chance of injury to your back.

Exercise Tip: In order to make lunges and squats more difficult, add dumbbells.

Beginner Level

Exercise	Sets	Repetitions
Reverse Lunges	1-2	10-12
Hamstring Blast	1-2	10-12
Hamstring Reach	1-2	10-12
Frog Lifts	1-2	10-12

Intermediate Level

Exercise	Sets	Repetitions
Squat Kicks	2-3	12-15
Lunge Ups	2-3	12-15
Single Legged Bridges	2-3	12-15
Frog Lifts	2-3	12-15

Advanced Level

Exercise	Sets	Repetitions
Squat Kicks	3-4	15-20
Frog Lifts	3-4	15-20
Single Legged Bridges	3-4	15-20
Hamstring Reaches	3-4	15-20
Lateral Lunges	3-4	15-20

Reverse Lunges

Targeted Muscles: quadriceps, glutes and hamstrings

Set Up: Stand with feet together, slight bend in knees with hands resting on hips or placed in front of body.

Action: With chest up and core tight, in a slow and controlled manner, step back with one leg, creating a wide stance between your front and back leg. Keep a slight bend in both knees without knees going over toes. Your back knee approaches the ground but never touches the ground. Hold for a count and push off back leg, bring back leg forward to starting position. Repeat movement until set is complete on one leg and then switch legs and repeat movement.

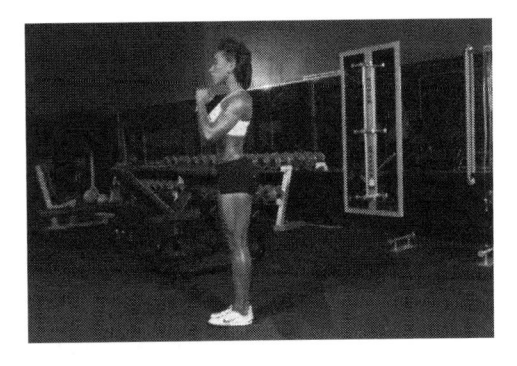

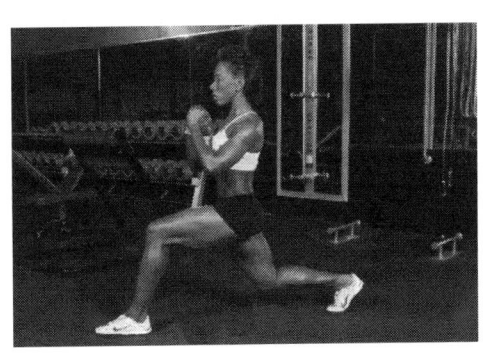

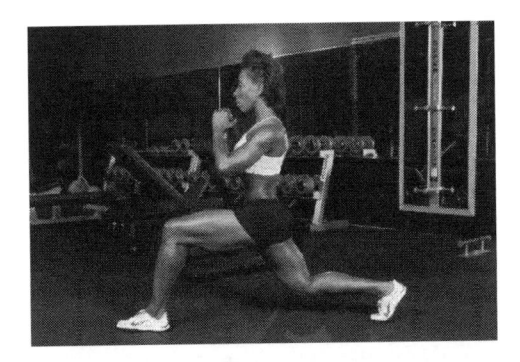

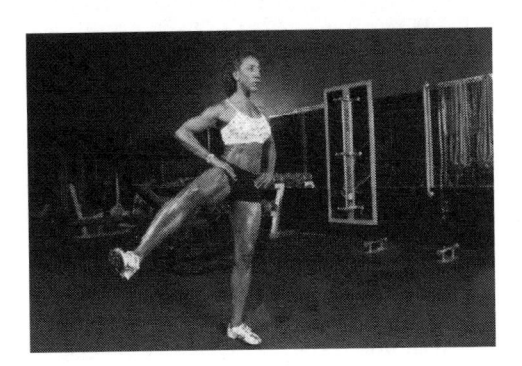

Reverse Lunge with Abductions

Targeted Muscles: quadriceps, glutes and hamstrings

Set Up: Stand with feet together, slight bend in knees, shoulders back, core engaged with hands resting on hips.

Action: In a slow and controlled manner, step back with one leg, creating a wide stance between your front and back leg. Keep a slight bend in both knees without knees going over toes. Your back knee approaches the ground but never touches the ground. Once in this position, hold for a count and then bring back leg forward to starting position.
From starting position, place sight bend in lead leg and move your leg away from the midline (middle) of your body. Hold for a count and then bring leg back to starting position. Switch legs and repeat movements with opposite leg.

Squat with Side Kick

Targeted Muscles: Glutes, hamstrings

Set Up: Stand with feet hip width apart, core tight and shoulder blades retracted

Action: In a slow and controlled manner, engage core and squat until your knees make a 90 degree angle. Hold squat for a count while maintaining proper form. Return completely from squat, shift weight onto right leg, and then kick out to the left side of your body. Bring leg back to ground, repeat squatting movement and perform kick with opposite leg.

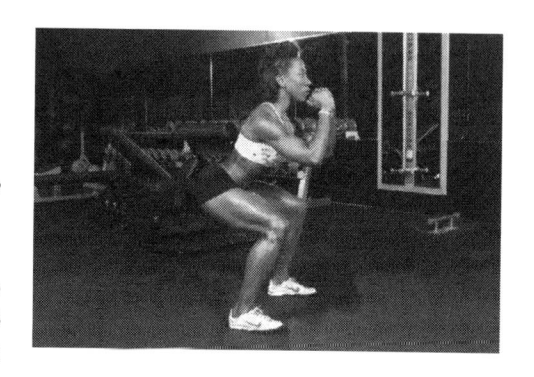

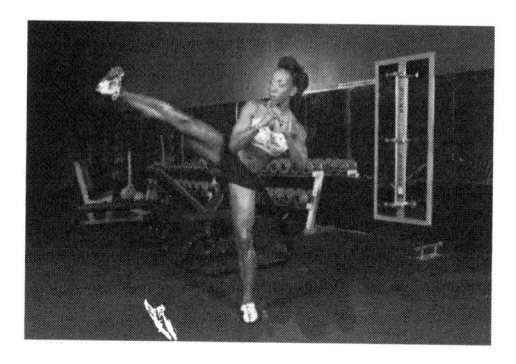

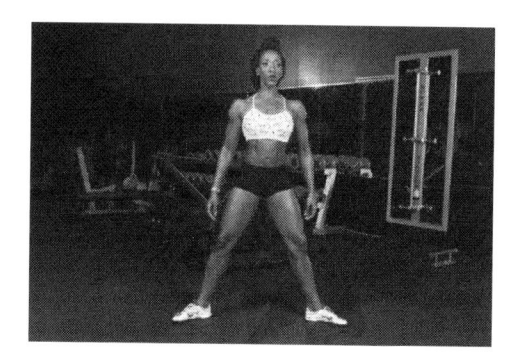

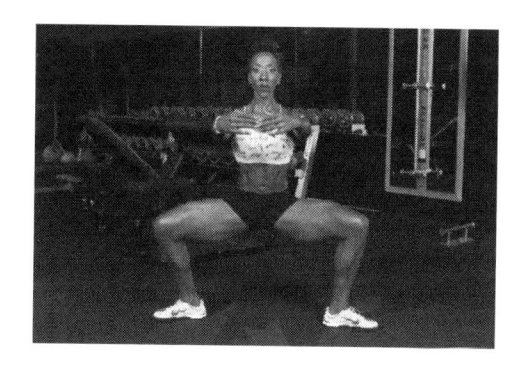

Plie Squats with Calf Raises

Targeted Muscles: calves, inner thighs, glutes

Set Up: Stand with feet wider than shoulder width apart, toes turned outward with core engaged and arms extended by body.

Action: In a slow and controlled manner, lower body until your thighs are parallel to the ground. Keep knees pointed in same direction as toes. Hold for a count and then return body back to starting position. While in an upward position, lift up on calves and perform a calve raise. Bring calves down. Repeat entire movement until set is complete.

*****Movement Tip**: Keep core contracted throughout entire movement. Do not allow knees to go over toes.

Lateral Lunges

Targeted Muscles: Glutes, hamstrings

Set Up: Place feet together or hip-width apart with your toes pointed directly forward. Shoulders back, core engaged and hands placed in front of body or positioned on hips.

Action: In a slow and controlled manner, lift your right leg and step to the side. Once your foot is fully planted, push your hips back and bend your right knee to lower into a lunge. Descend until your right thigh is about parallel to the floor and then extend your hips and knee to come back up.
Return your right foot to the starting position and then perform the next repetition, stepping to the side with your left foot. Continue this back and forth movement pattern until you complete set.

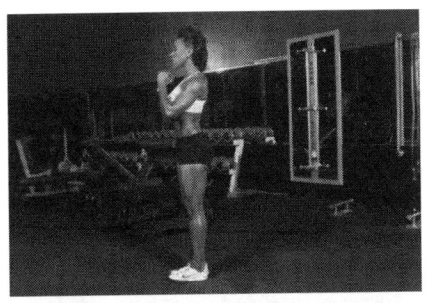

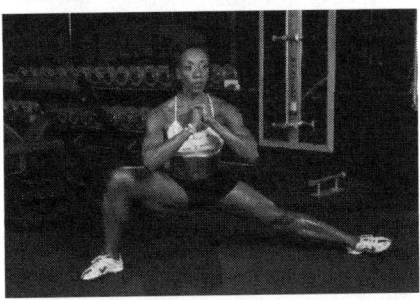

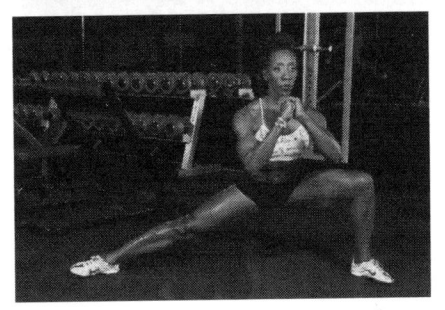

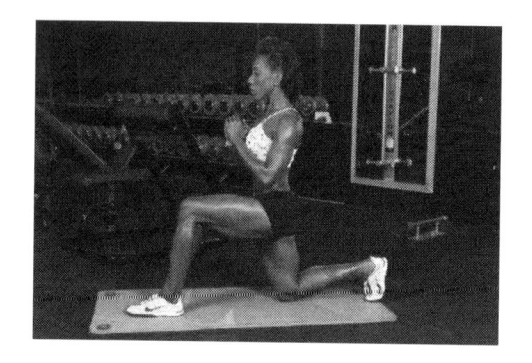

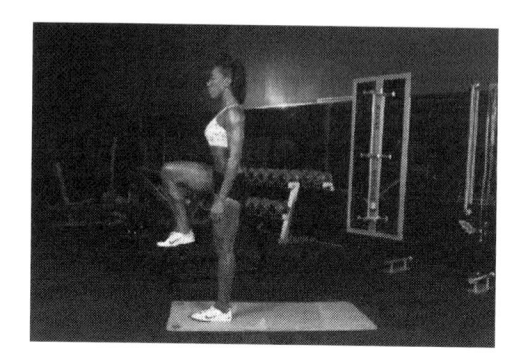

Lunge Ups

Targeted Muscles: glutes, thighs (quadriceps) & hamstrings

Set Up: Begin with body in a stationary lunge position, right leg back, core engaged with hands positioned in front of body or on hips.

Action: In a slow and controlled manner, push off back leg, bringing body into an upward position shifting weight from back leg to front left leg. Hold body in this position for a count and then slowly lower right leg back to starting position. Repeat movement pattern on right leg until set is complete and then switch legs and repeat movement until set is complete.

Single-Legged Bridge

Targeted Muscle: glutes, hamstrings

Set Up: Lie on your back with both feet placed on the ground knees bent, with arms extended by your side.

Action: In a slow and controlled manner, slowly lift right leg off ground, while bridging up on left leg by squeezing your glutes and hamstrings. Hold body in this position for a count and then slowly lower left hip and right leg. Switch legs and repeat movement pattern on the opposite side of your body until set is complete.

*****Modified Version**: Keep both feet on ground, and then bridge up.

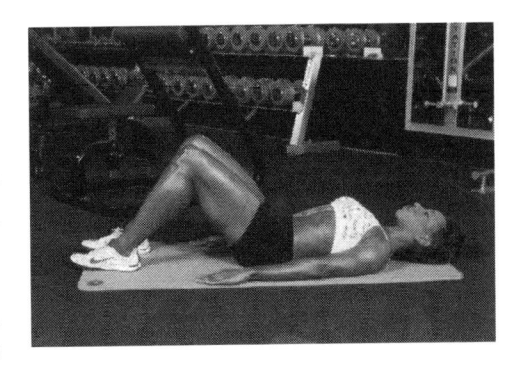

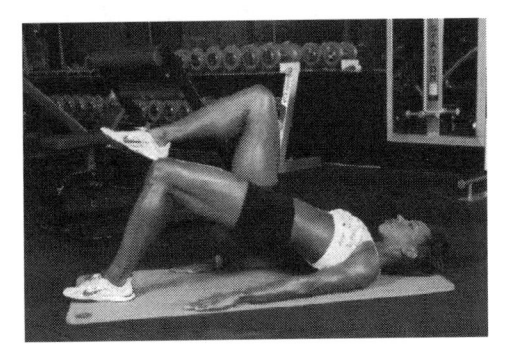

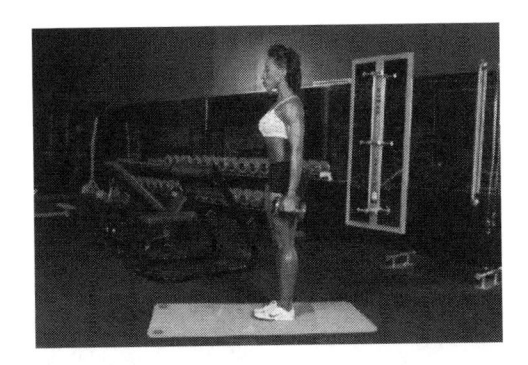

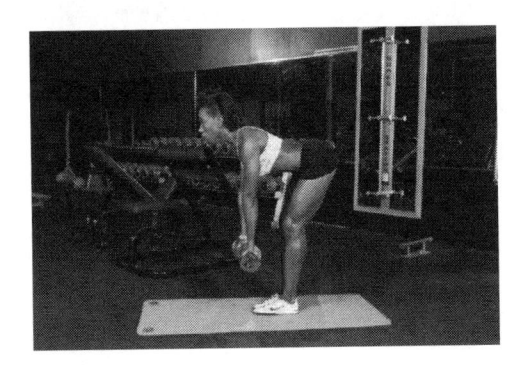

Hamstring Reach

Targeted Muscles: glutes, hamstrings

Set Up: Stand with feet together, slight bend in knees. Arms extended by your side with hands in a neutral position (palms facing inwards towards your body).

Action: While maintaining a slight bend in knees and core engaged, in a slow and controlled manner, bring torso forward reaching dumbbells towards ground and pushing hips back. Hold for a count and then return body back to starting position. Repeat movement until set is complete.

Frog Lifts

Targeted Muscles: glutes, hamstrings

Set Up: Roll forward on stability ball until hips are positioned midway on ball, legs spread apart forming a "V," feet touching ground with arms positioned shoulder width apart.

Action: While keeping legs in "V" position, in a slow and controlled manner, squeeze glutes and move legs in an upward movement towards the ceiling. Hold for a count and then bring legs back to starting position. Repeat movement until set is complete.

*Movement Tip: Keep a slight bend in elbows throughout entire movement. Keep head forward in a neutral position.

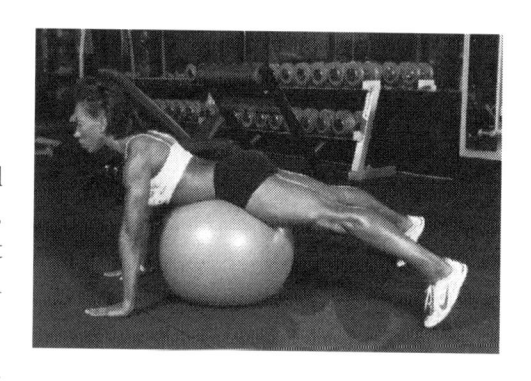

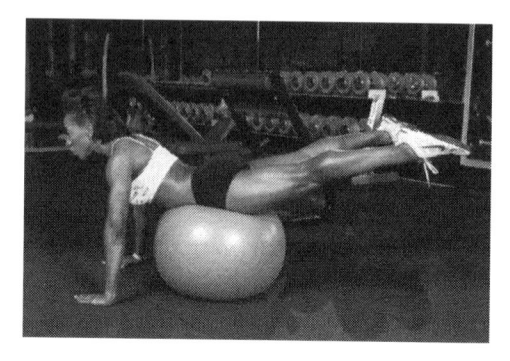

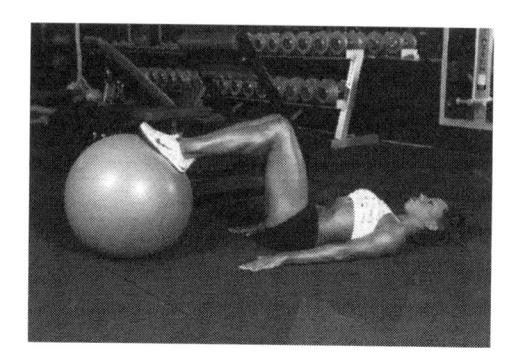

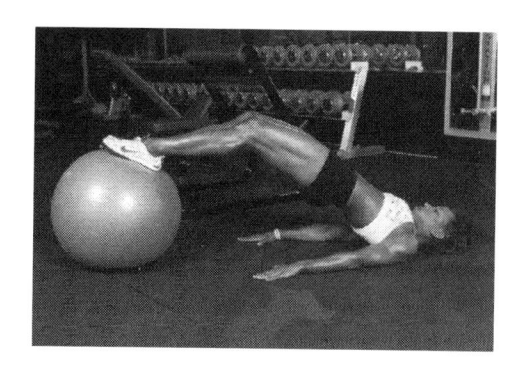

Hamstring Blast

Targeted Muscles: hamstrings, glutes

Set Up: Lay on your back with knees bent, feet flat on stability ball, arms resting near body with palms in a downward position.

Action: In a slow and controlled manner, create an arc movement by pressing feet against ball and lifting hips off ground. Hold for a count and then return body back to starting position. Repeat movement until set is complete.

CHANGING THE NORM

Curtsy Lunge

Targeted Muscle: quads, glutes, hamstrings

Set Up: Stand with right leg in front and left leg positioned diagonally behind right leg. Slight bend in knees, with hands rested on hips.

Action: In a slow and controlled manner, bend both knees until your thigh is parallel to the ground. Your back knees approaches, but never touches the ground. Hold for a count and then return body back to starting position. Repeat movement until set is complete and then switch front and back legs, repeat movement with opposite stance until set is complete.

*****Movement Tip**: Make sure knee doesn't go past toes. Keep body in proper alignment with core contracted throughout entire movement.

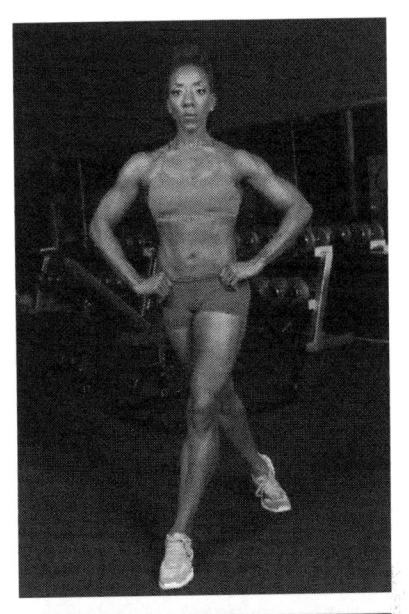

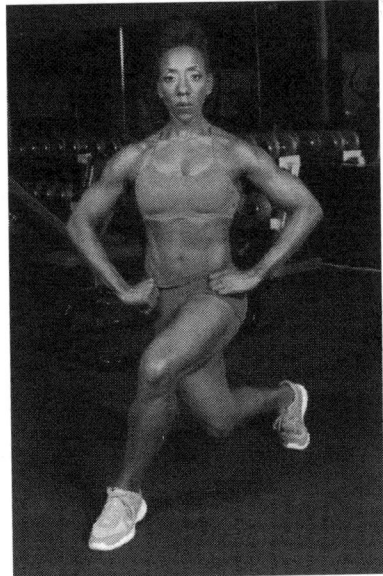

FIT JEWEL

You can't spot reduce to lose weight in a particular part of your legs! You can train smart, consistently and consume healthy well-balanced meals to assist you in losing weight in your legs and your entire body.

CHANGING THE NORM

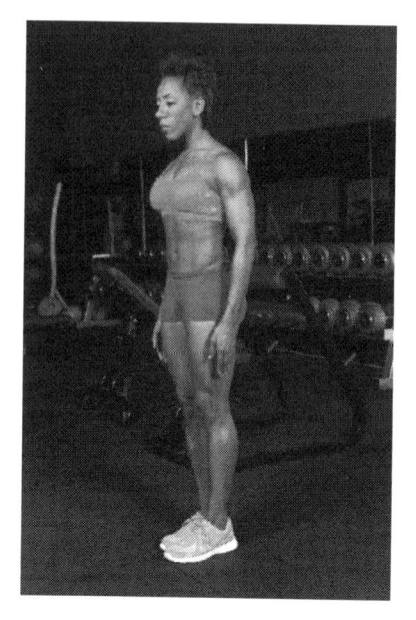

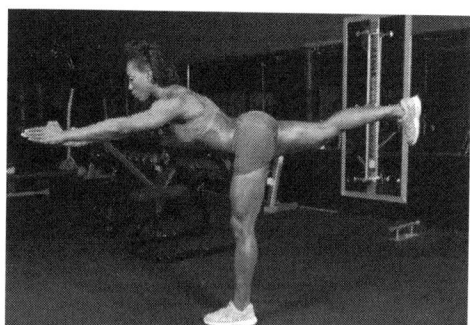

Tick Tocks

Targeted Muscle: glutes, quads (thighs) and hamstrings

Set Up: Stand with feet together, slight bend in knees, arms by your side.

Action: While contracting core, in a slow and controlled manner, bring torso forward reaching both arms in front of body while lifting right leg off the ground. Keep eyes forward and locate a focal point in order to maintain balance. Hold body in this position for a count and then bring body back to starting position. Repeat movement and switch legs. Repeat movement pattern until set is complete.

FIT JEWEL

Squat, lunge and bridge for tighter and firmer legs, but don't forget clean eating and regular cardio to help you shed unwanted body fat from your legs. Don't let your hard work go to waste!

Standing Hip Abductions

Targeted Muscles: abductors, glutes

Set Up: Stand with feet together, slight bend in knees. Hands placed on hips or in front of your body.

Action: With slight bend in knee, in a slow and controlled manner, lift leg off ground away from the mid-line or middle of body with knee pointing downward. Keep bend in opposite leg. Hold for a count and then return leg back to starting position. Repeat movement and then switch leg and repeat movement until set is complete with opposite leg.

***Movement Tip**: While lifting leg, keep core tight to avoid a shift of weight on supporting leg. If you lack balance or core strength, find an object to hold onto for support.

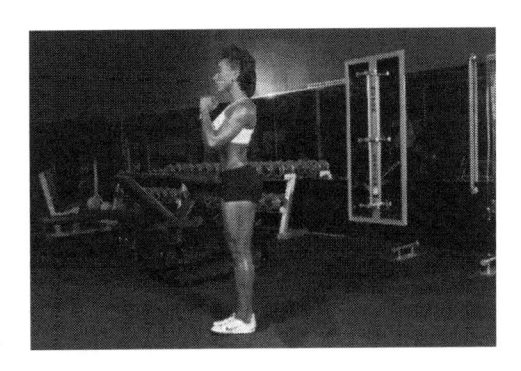

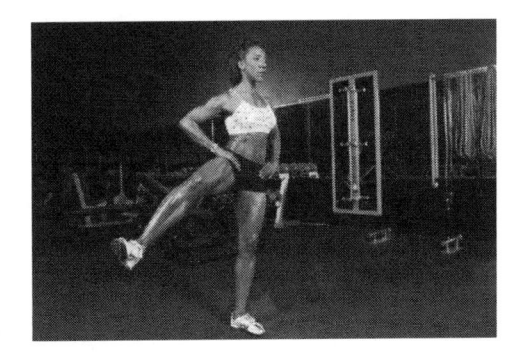

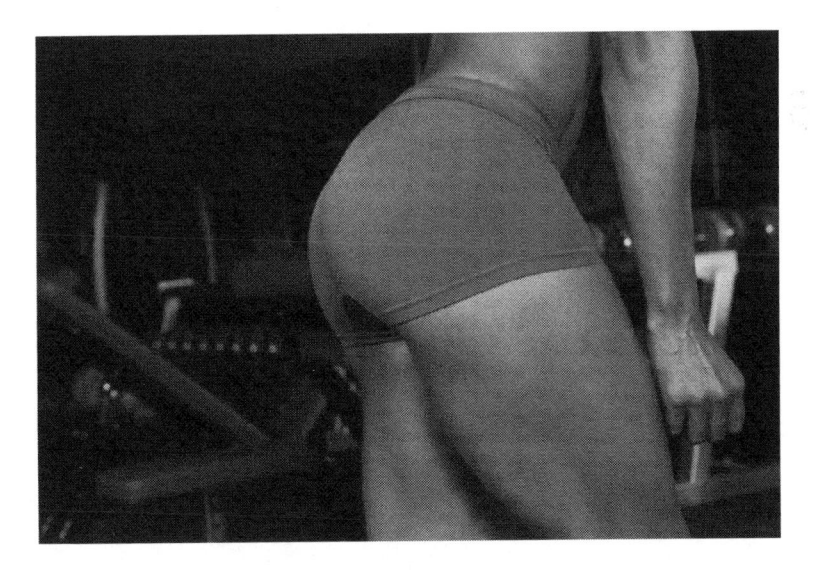

GOT CURVES?

Abdominal Exercises

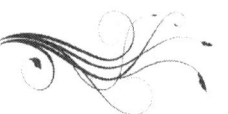

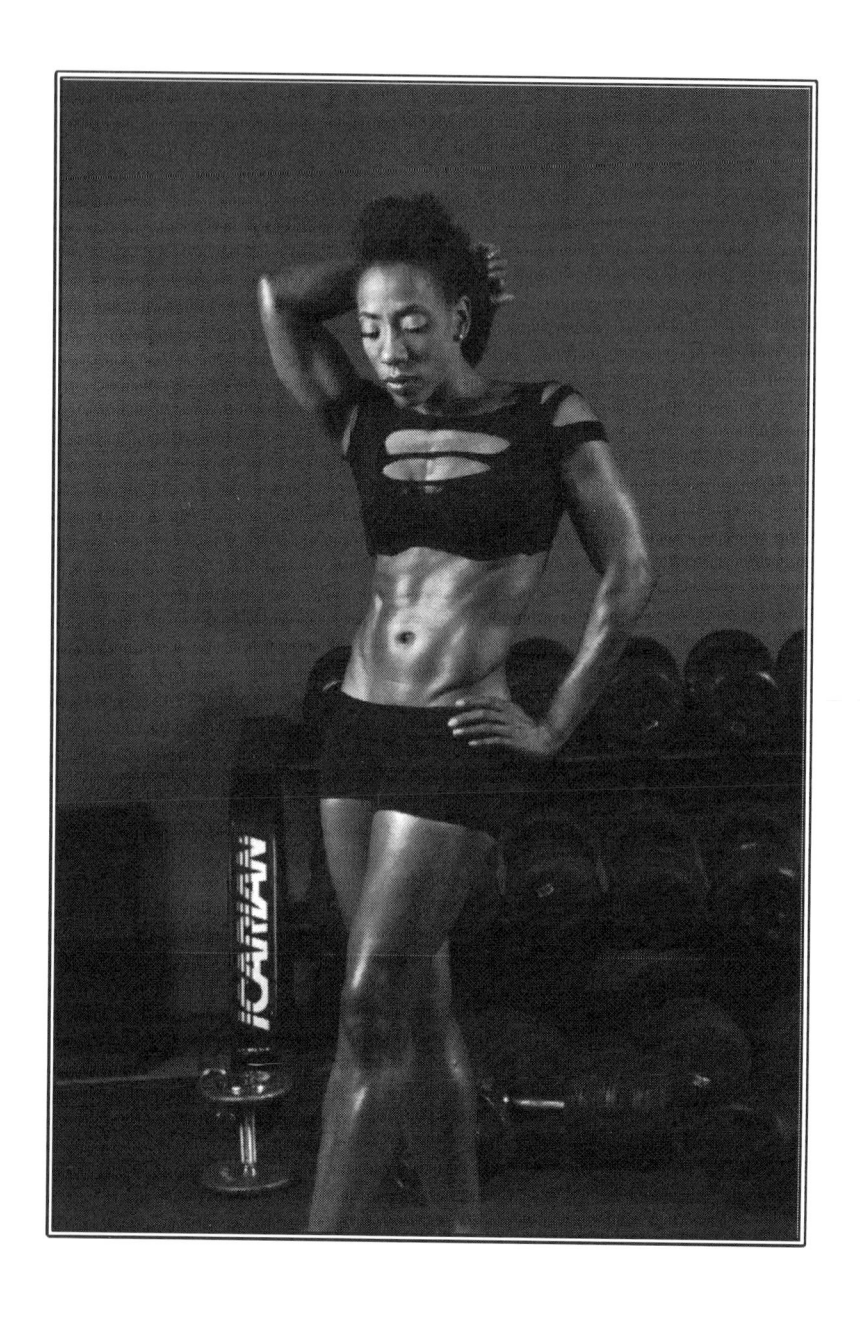

CHANGING THE NORM

A Stronger Core, A Stronger You

Your core or abdominal muscles are one of the most important muscle groups in the entire body. Every movement performed requires core stabilization and strength. For some women, this is a challenging area to tone and strengthen. Some women have given birth and as a result have weakened core muscles. On the other hand, some women have jobs that require long hours of sitting and as a result, their core muscles have been weakened and they experience low back pain. Regardless of your profession or whether you are a mother, having a strong core is essential to all of your movements.

Therefore the exercises on the following pages will help you create a more toned and strong core.

A STRONGER CORE = BETTER POSTURE

Abdominal Exercises

Movement Tip: Keep core contracted while performing each exercise. This will keep body aligned and lessen the chance of injury to your back.

Beginner Level

Exercise	Sets	Repetitions
Knee Taps	2	8-10
Physio-ball reverse knees	2	8-10
Ropes	2	8-10
Walk-Ups	2	8-10

Intermediate Level

Exercise	Sets	Repetitions
Russian Twists with Layout	2-3	12-15
Med-ball Oblique Twists	2-3	12-15
Hanging Abdominal Raises	2-3	12-15
Ropes	2-3	12-15

Advanced Level

Exercise	Sets	Repetitions
Russian Twists with Layout	3-4	15-20
Med-ball Oblique Twists	3-4	15-20
Hanging Abdominal Raises	3-4	15-20
Ropes	3-4	15-20

CHANGING THE NORM

Knee Taps

Targeted Muscles: oblique's

Set Up: Begin with feet placed shoulder width apart, slight bend in knees with arms extended overhead while holding medicine ball.

Action: In a slow and controlled manner, contract core and bring right elbow and right knee together, hold for a count. Return to starting position. Repeat movement until set is complete. Switch arm and leg and then repeat movement until set is complete.

*****Movement Tip**: Keep slight bend in knees throughout entire movement.

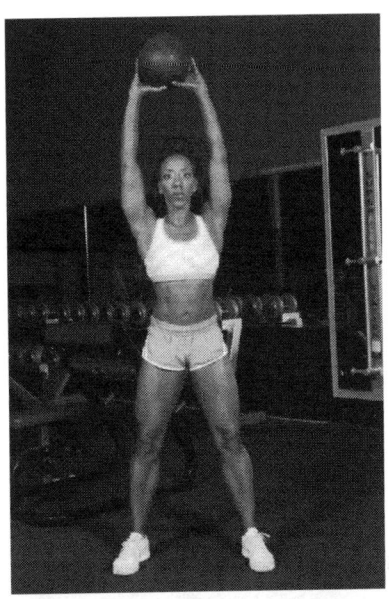

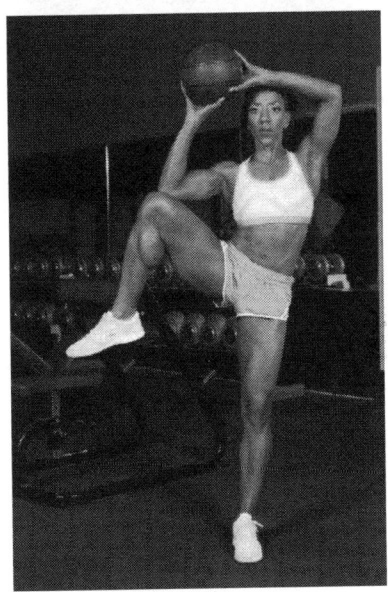

FIT JEWEL

It is essential to remember that although you may strengthen and tone your abdominal muscles with exercise, in order to see your abs, you have to burn the fat surrounding your abs by incorporating healthy well-balanced meals and cardio.

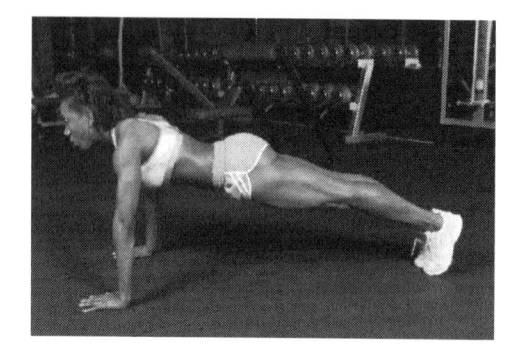

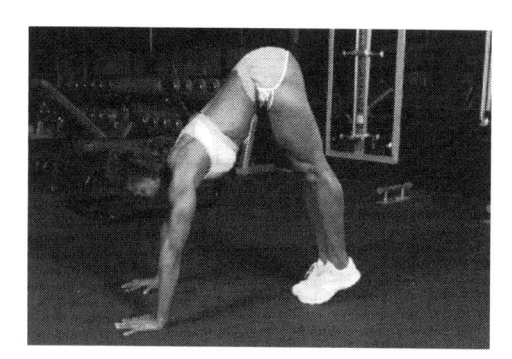

Walk-Ups

Targeted Muscles: abdominals

Set Up: Begin in a push up position, arms shoulder width apart with slight bend in elbows, core tight, lower body in a straight line.

Action: In a slow and controlled manner, step backwards with your hands until your body is in a "V" position. Hold position for a count and then slowly bring body down by moving hands forwards. Repeat movement until set is complete.

***Movement Tip**: Only go as far as your natural range of motion will allow.

Movement Tip:

This is an Advanced Move, Only Perform if Your Body Allows!

Russian Twists with Layout

Targeted Muscles: abdominals, oblique's

Set Up: Place body on mat with feet flat on ground, knees bent, chest up while arms are bent holding medicine ball.

Action: In a slow and controlled manner, bring feet off mat around 2- 4 inches. Once stabilized, rotate torso from one side to the other side of the body. After rotation, return torso to starting position, while in this position extend arms overhead and release legs straight in front of your body. Hold for a count and then repeat movement until set is complete.

*****Modified Version**: Keep feet on ground when rotating and do not perform layout.

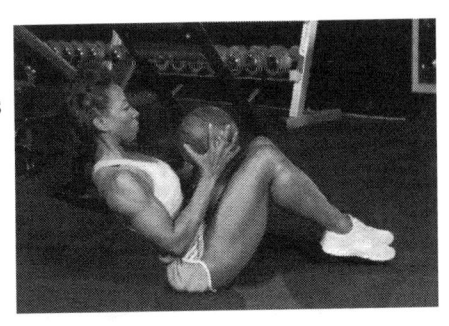

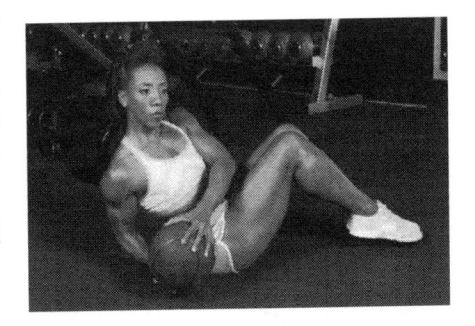

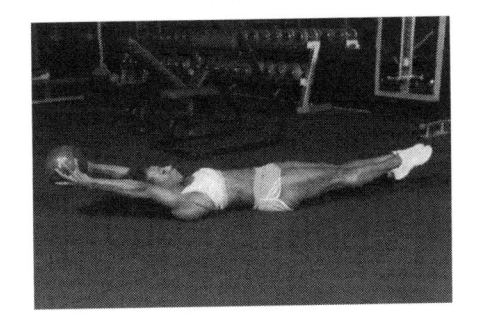

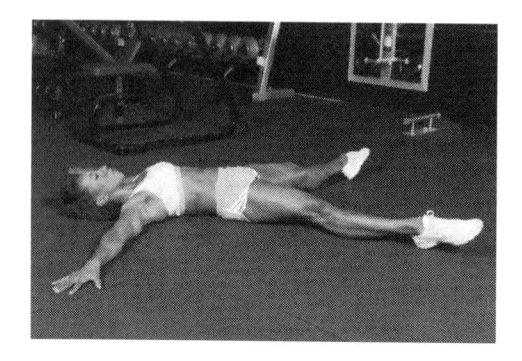

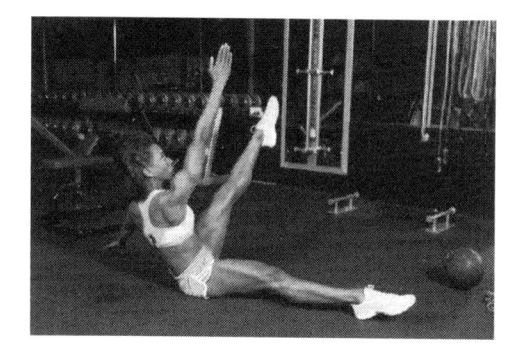

Switch-n-Reach

Targeted Muscles: oblique's

Set Up: Lie down on a mat with body in a jumping jack position. Arms and legs form an "X".
Action: In a slow and controlled manner, bring right arm towards left leg. Hold for a count and then bring body back to staring position. From starting position, switch arm and leg and repeat movement until set is complete.
Movement Tip: Only lift arm and leg within natural range of motion.
*Modified Version: Keep upper body in same position with legs placed on ground. Instead of bringing arm and leg together, reach opposite arm towards opposite leg by slightly lifting shoulder off mat.

Pike Holds

Targeted Muscles: abdominals

Set Up: In a slow and controlled manner, roll body forward on stability ball until shins rest on ball. Hands are positioned shoulder width apart, core tight and legs in a straight line.

Action: With a slight bend in elbows, in a slow and controlled manner, slowly draw in stomach and lift body into a pike position creating a "V." Hold for a count and then slowly bring body back to starting position. Repeat movement until set is complete.

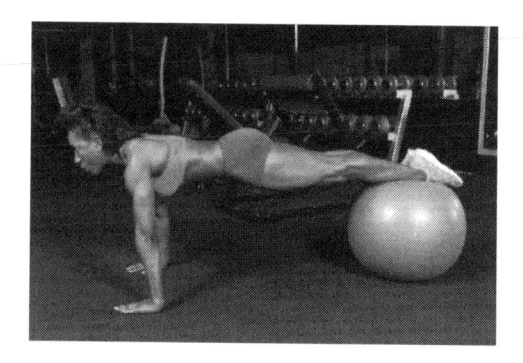

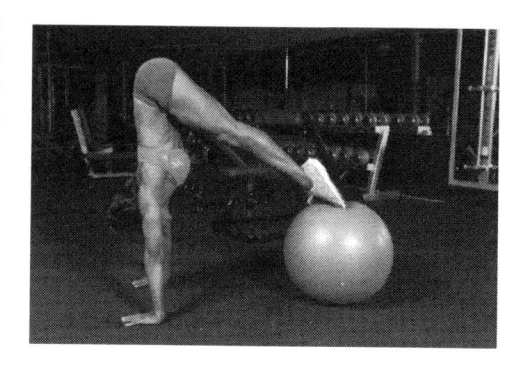

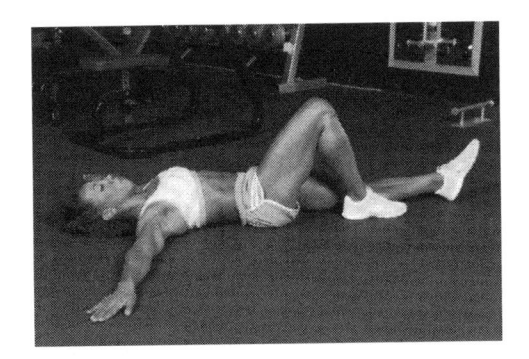

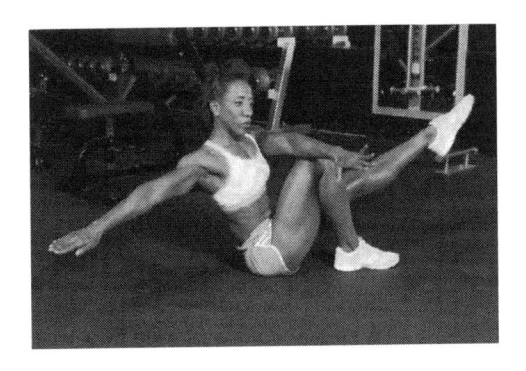

Windmills

Targeted Muscles: abdominals, oblique's

Set Up: While lying on your back, extend both arms out to the side of your body, with left leg fully extended and right knee bent with foot on floor.

Action: In a slow and controlled manner lift upper body off ground in a rotational movement, reaching left arms towards right knee, while right foot lifts off ground. Hold for a count and rotate body back to starting position. Perform movement until set is complete. Switch legs and repeat entire movement on opposite side.

Physio-ball Reverse Knees

Targeted Muscles: abdominals

Set Up: While lying on your back, place physio-ball in between your legs, slightly squeezing your thigh muscles to keep the ball stabilized. Feet are at in a flexed position on ground.

Action: In a slow and controlled manner, engage core and bring feet off ground and knees towards upper body. Hold for a count and slowly bring feet back to ground without allowing feet to fully rest on ground. Repeat movement until set is completed.

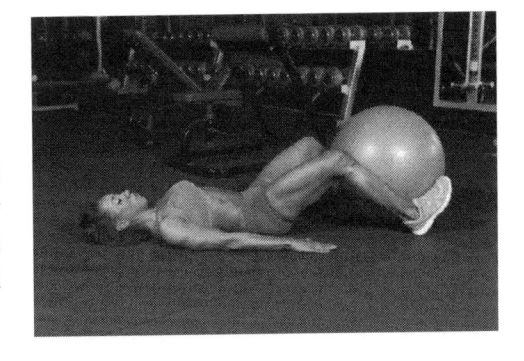

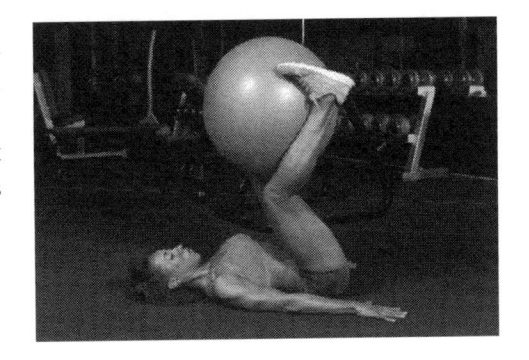

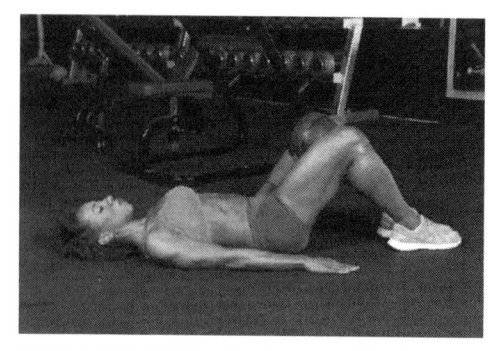

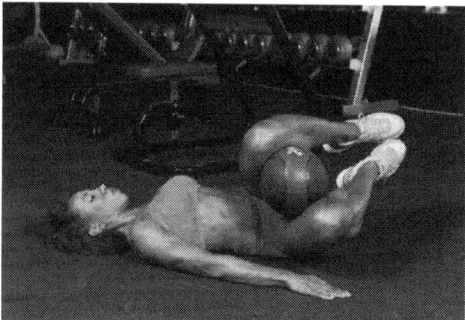

Med-ball Oblique Twists

Targeted Muscles: abdominals, oblique's

Set up: While lying on your back, with arms extended on ground next to body, knees bent, place medicine ball between thigh muscles, with feet flat on ground.

Action: In a slow and controlled manner, lift feet off ground and rotate hips and knees towards the side of your body. Hold for a count and then bring legs back to the middle of your body and rotate them in the opposite direction and hold for a count. Repeat this movement pattern until set is complete.

Movement tip: Try to keep shoulders on ground when rotating body from side to side. If you can't properly execute movement with medicine ball, remove medicine ball and perform movement without it.

Ropes

Targeted Muscles: abdominals

Set Up: Lay on ground with knees bent, feet flat on floor and arms extended over your head, with one arm staggered over the other.

Action: In a slow and controlled manner engage your core and pretend your hands are climbing up a rope, one hand at a time. Once body is completely off the floor, hold for a count and then slowly reverse your hands climbing back down the rope as your torso returns back to the ground. Repeat movement until set is completed.

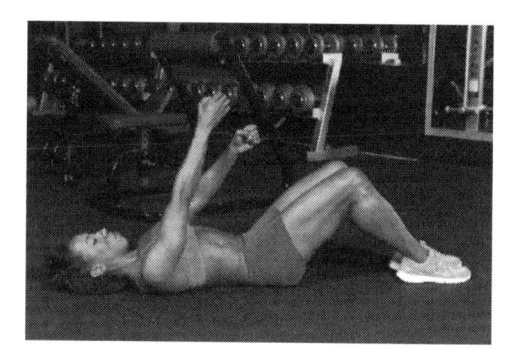

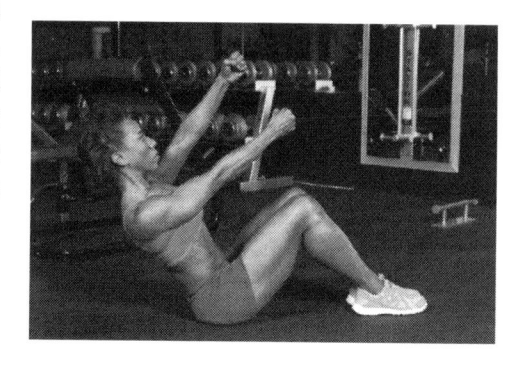

Hanging Abdominal Raises

Targeted Muscles: abdominals

Set Up: In a slow and controlled manner, jump up or use a bench to grasp and hang from a high bar (Universal Machine) with hands positioned slightly wider than shoulder width apart with an overhand grip, core engaged and body stabilized.

Action: In a slow and controlled manner, slowly raise legs by flexing hips and knees until hips are completely flexed or knees are well above hips. Hold for a count and then slowly return hips and knees to starting position. Repeat movement until set is completed.

Movement tip: When performing this movement do not allow body to swing back and forth. Keep core engaged throughout entire movement and keep slight bend in elbows while hanging from bar.

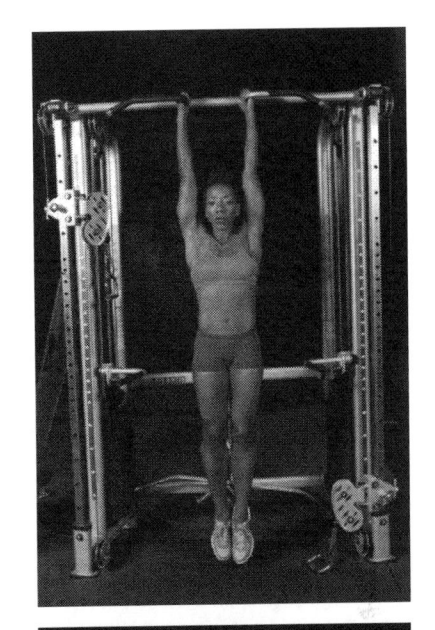

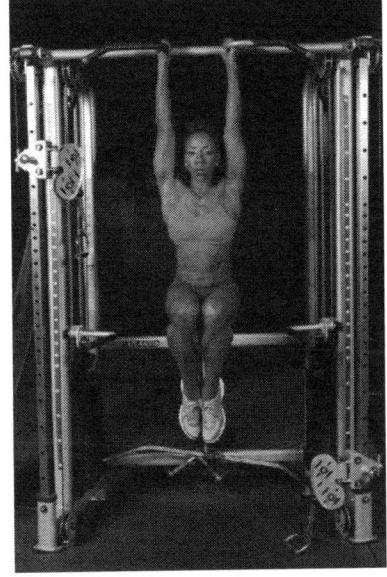

Movement Tip:
Keep Your Eyes Forward, This Will Help With Balance!

Curve Sculpting Exercise Tracking Sheet

Use the following sheet to track your exercises, rank your intensity levels and mental preparedness for each workout.

Make copies and place into a binder to create your own fitness training log.

Date:

Exercise	Sets	Repetitions	Rest Time

Mental Fit:

Having a positive attitude about your workout can produce great results. Therefore, before you start your workout, take time to gauge your mental preparation.

Rank your mindset for your workout:
1. I am extremely focused.
2. I am tired, but no more excuses.
3. I will do it because I have to.
4. I am excited about seeing my body change.

Intensity Level:

The amount of effort you put into your workout will determine your overall results.

Rank the amount of effort you put into your workout.
1. I gave 100% - no slacking.
2. I could have pushed harder.
3. I wasn't excited about the workout, but gave it all I had.

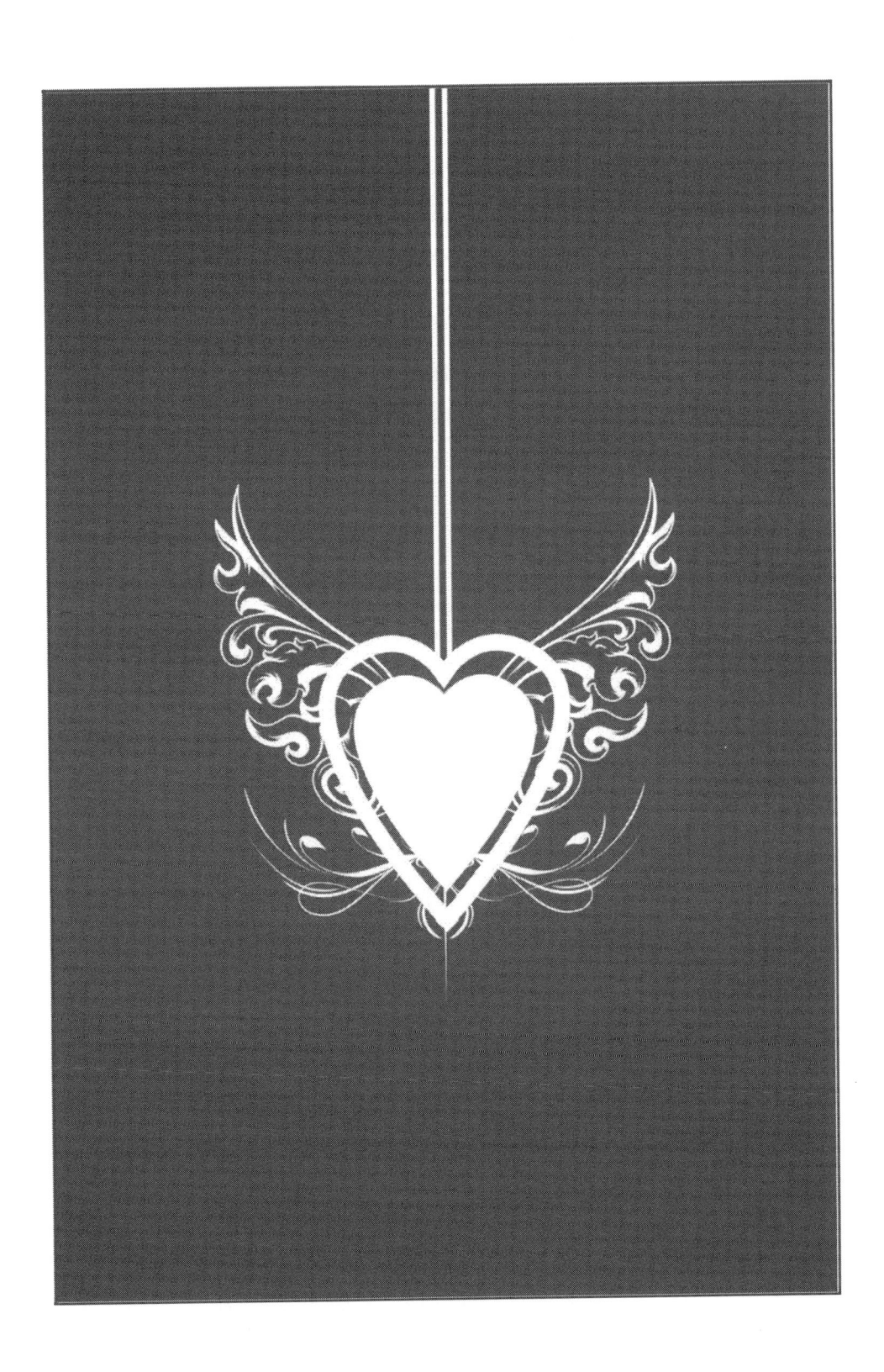

Chapter 29

From my HEART to yours

What an Amazing Accomplishment!

As you end with this chapter, it is my hope that something you read has helped you see yourself, your health and your body in a different light.

Yes, you're smart, you're beautiful and creative, however, the question I want you to always ask yourself is " Are you healthy"? If the answer to this question is no, I desire for you to ask yourself why! Understanding your why, will put you on a path to honesty and change, if that's the place you desire to go!

As you start or continue your health and fitness journey, take each day to continually work on becoming a better version of yourself. It is essential to remember that change does not occur overnight; it's a gradual and sometimes slow, yet rewarding process. Therefore be patient with yourself and allow time for personal growth and physical changes.

To remain positive and focused, continue creating a support system and don't be afraid to ask for help when you need it. Yes, I know you're a "STRONG, BEAUTIFUL BLACK WOMAN", but you can let your hair down and just be you sometimes. I want to once again encourage you to ask for help when you need it and refuse to allow life to box you in the "NORM" category any longer!

Although I am not with you in person, I carry your struggles and successes in my heart. On the days when you feel alone, remember there are millions of other African American women who feel the same way you do.

Break your "NORMS" and let your light shine so bright that the world mistakes you for a star.

I look forward to hearing what you have discovered about yourself, and how you are transforming your mind and body!

Please e-mail me at laticiaactionjackson@gmail.com and share your personal story.

Remember, failure is never an option!

God Bless You

Laticia "Action" Jackson ~ **Stay fit, Stay true, Stay you!**

About the Author
Laticia " Action" Jackson

Health and Fitness Expert Laticia "Action" Jackson has been called one of the most energetic and passionate personalities in the health promotion, wellness and fitness industry both nationally and globally!

Her successful career as 2008 Fitness Olympian and 3-Time State National Physique Committee Fitness Champion has provided her with the opportunity to be featured in over 20 national and international fitness, health and wellness magazines.

With an academic success that includes a Master's Degree in Public Health, B.S. Degree in Exercise Physiology, Certified Master Level Personal Trainer, Certified Weight Loss Counselor, Certified Corporate Wellness Coach and Certified Lifestyle Coach, it has been proven that Laticia "Action" Jackson has the knowledge, skills and ability to help improve health outcomes for individuals and groups. To date "Action" Jackson has helped to improve the health outcomes of thousands, assisted companies in creating healthier work environments and has provided educational insight and support to high-risk communities.

Action Jackson's mission to empower individuals to take control of their lives by first taking control of their health has led her to being featured as the go-to health and fitness expert for television stations such as C.W. 31, Fox 45/ ABC 22, WEAR 3, Blab T.V. and many more.

She's often called upon from national organizations such as the American Heart Association, American Diabetes Association and The American Cancer Society to use her dynamic personality and expertise for nation-wide health promotion events.

Why stop there?

"Action" Jackson is a Veteran of the U.S.A.F., member of Delta Sigma Theta Sorority Inc. and a survivor of domestic violence who's become an domestic violence advocate. Learn more about Action Jackson and her additional books, products and services by visiting her website at www.laticiaactionjackson.com.

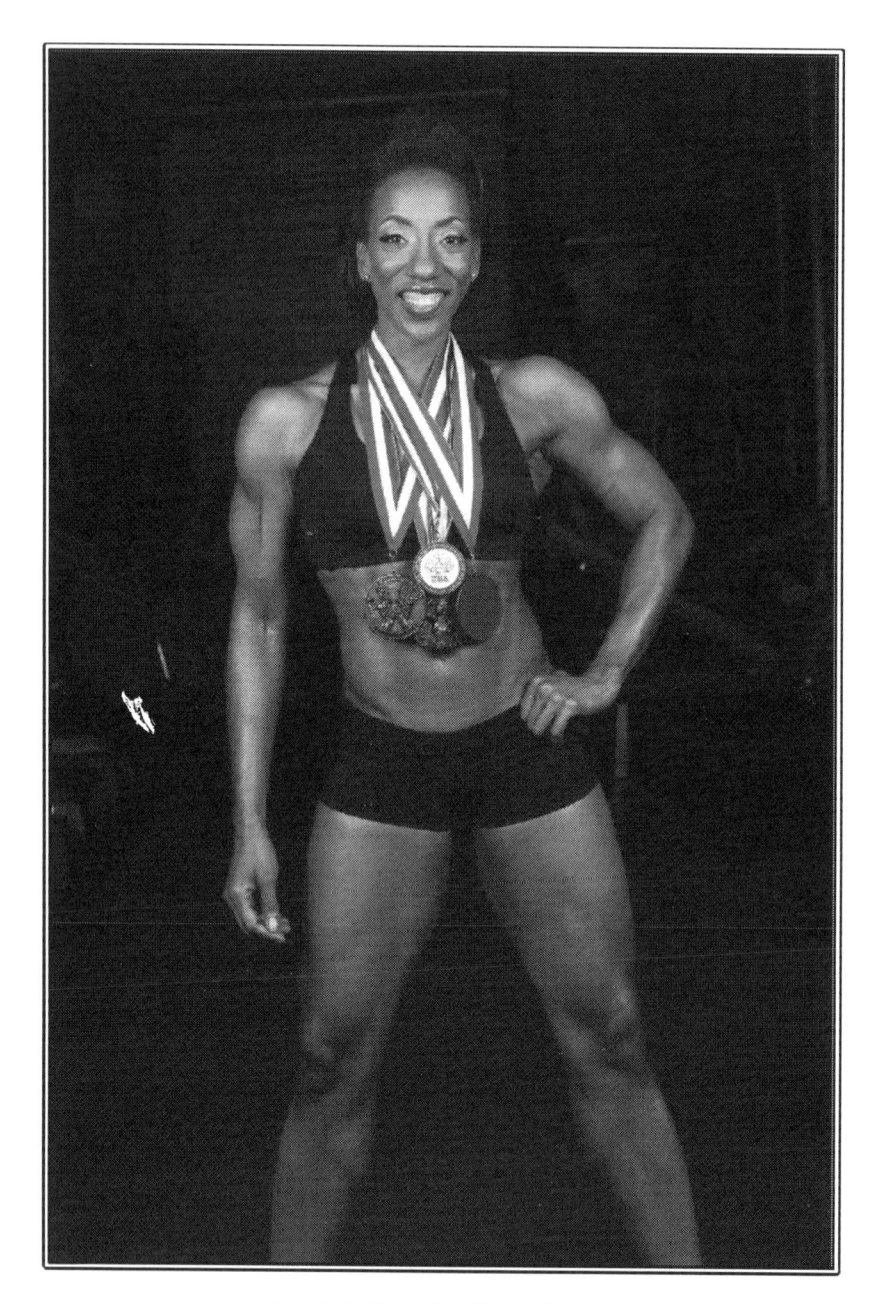

Laticia "Action" Jackson

2008 Fitness Olympian/ 3-Time NPC Fitness Champion

Index

A

Abduction, 169
Accomplishments, 31
Adduction, 169
Afraid, 44, 52, 59, 107, 166, 175, 178, 182, 192, 242
Age, 29, 30, 31, 32, 69, 145, 164, 183, 191
Amino acids, 68, 70, 71
Anorexia, 64
Anterior Shoulder Stretch, 185
Atrophy, 169

B

Bacteria, 176
Beef, 72, 73
BMI, 145, 146, 147, 150
Body composition, 142
Breakfast, 96, 97, 104
Budget, 101, 103
Bulimia, 64

C

Calf Stretch, 187
Carbohydrate, 71, 82, 83, 85, 92, 93, 97, 173
Carbohydrates, 68, 81, 82, 84, 85, 92, 93, 94, 99, 105, 106, 108, 109, 110
Carbohydrates, 81, 82, 85, 92
Cardio, 136, 137, 152, 163, 167, 172, 176, 177, 178, 179, 181
Cardiovascular, 72, 135, 136, 137, 138, 139, 147, 149, 150, 151, 159, 161, 163, 164, 167, 178, 188, 189
Cardiovascular, 136, 137, 138, 159, 161, 163, 167, 169
Chest, 36, 156, 157, 180, 185, 186
Chicken, 110
Circuit training, 159

Clip Coupons, 102
Commitment, 28, 30, 52
Complex, 82, 83, 92, 93, 97, 99, 116, 173
Complex carbohydrates, 82
Concentric, 169
Condiments, 99
Consistency, 143, 158
Core, 147, 156, 162, 171, 180, 181, 185, 192, 193, 197, 200, 205, 210, 220, 231, 232
Core Shoulder Lifts, 200

D

Desire, 69, 84, 136, 137, 151, 159, 160, 178
Dinner, 48, 104, 107
Dreams, 41, 51

E

Eating, 101
Eccentric, 169
Ectomorph, 134, 136, 137
Eggs, 106
Elbow extension, 169
Elbow flexion, 169
Emotional eating, 97
Endomorph, 134, 136
Energy, 81, 82, 83, 92, 96, 107, 137, 145, 165, 166
Exercise Tracking Sheet, 240
Extension, 169
Extensions, 169

F

F.I.T.T. model, 184
Fat, 70, 71, 74, 75, 76, 77, 78, 79, 81, 89, 92, 97, 98, 99, 105, 106, 108,

109, 110, 112, 138, 139, 141, 142, 143, 144, 145, 163, 167, 219
Fitness goals, 31, 49, 93, 141, 171
Fitness training level, 188
Fitness Training Level, 189
Flexibility, 169
Flexion, 169, 170
Free weights, 161,
162 Frog Lifts, 220
Front Shoulder Raises, 158, 200
Full body training, 157, 158

G

Giant set, 159
Girth measurements, 143
Gluteal (buttocks) Stretch,
186 Glutes, 219
Glycemic Index, 85, 86,
90 Grocery, 102
Gym, 28, 71, 143, 152, 158, 171, 172, 173, 174, 175, 176, 178

H

Hamstring Blast, 220
Hamstring Reach, 220
Hamstring Reaches, 220
Hamstring Stretch, 186
Hamstring Stretch (Lying Down), 186 Hamstring Stretch (Standing), 186 Hanging Abdominal Raises, 232
Health, 103
Healthier, 103
Healthy, 101, 103
Healthy eating, 72
Heart, 3, 34, 36, 37, 53, 74, 75, 76, 77, 81, 98, 138, 149, 159, 163, 164, 170, 173
Heart disease, 34, 36, 37, 74, 75, 76 Heart Disease, 36
Heart healthy, 36
Hypertrophy, 169

I

Ingredient labels, 61, 62, 76
Interval training, 160, 177, 178
Intrinsically motivated, 153

K

Knee Taps, 232
Kneeling Physio-ball Curls, 205

L

Lateral, 158, 159, 169, 180, 200, 220
Lifestyle, 103
Lunch, 72, 107
Lunge Ups, 220

M

Maximum heart rate,
170 Meal, 102
Measurements, 139, 141, 142, 143, 144, 145, 146, 150, 151
Med-ball Oblique Twists, 232
Menu Planning Sheet, 125
Mesomorph, 134, 136
Monounsaturated, 74, 75 Muscle group, 137, 156, 158, 159
Muscles, 68, 151, 155, 156, 157, 158, 165, 167, 168, 184, 231
Muscular Endurance, 163, 170
Muscular Strength, 163, 170

N

Negative attitudes, 52 Nutrients, 62, 63, 66, 68, 99, 107 Nutrition facts, 62, 63, 98 Nutrition label, 61, 63, 70 Nutritional content, 104
Nuts, 77

CHANGING THE NORM

O

Obesity, 74, 98
One-Arm Med Ball Pushups, 192, 193
One-Arm Row, 197
Outlets, 102
Overwhelming, 103

P

Physio-ball Chest Press, 192
Physio-ball Pushups, 192, 193
Physio-ball reverse knees, 232
Physio-ball Triceps Pushups, 210
Polyunsaturated fat, 74, 75
Polyunsaturated fats, 77 Principle of Adaptation, 168 Principle of Individual Differences, 168
Principle of Overload, 169
Principle of Progression, 168
Principle of Specificity, 168
Principle of Use/Disuse, 168
Processed foods, 81, 83
Proper breathing, 156
Protein, 68, 69, 70, 71, 72, 84, 92, 105, 106, 108, 109, 110, 114, 116, 173
Protein, 68, 69, 70, 72
Proteins, 68, 71
Pyramid Pushups, 210

Q

Quadriceps (front part of leg) Stretch, 187

R

Range of motion, 183 Rear Shoulder Raises, 200
Repetition, 170
Resistance Band Extensions, 210
Resistance Bands Curls, 205
Resistance training, 138, 152, 156, 160, 161, 167, 168, 179, 183, 188, 189, 191

Respiratory, 170
Reverse Lunges, 220
Ropes, 232
Russian Twists with Layout, 232

S

Saturated fat, 76, 79
Seated Overhead Triceps Extensions, 210
Seated Resistance Band Rows, 197 Set, 139, 140, 158, 159, 170, 193 Shoulder Rolls, 185
Simple sugars, 82, 83, 84, 99
Single Legged Bridges, 220
Single-Legged Bicep Curls, 205
Single-Legged Chest Press, 192
Snacks, 59, 71, 76, 79, 84, 97, 98
Sodium, 62, 98, 99, 105, 106
Split Stance Hammer Curls, 205
Split training, 156, 157, 158 Split training, 156, 157
Squat Kicks, 220
Standing Triceps Kickbacks, 210
Super setting, 158

T

Thoughts, 38, 39, 43
Training, 68, 71, 127, 134, 137, 139, 145, 150, 153, 154, 155, 156, 157, 158, 159, 160, 161, 163, 165, 166, 167, 168, 169, 171, 173, 177, 178, 183, 188, 189, 240
Trans fats, 74, 75, 76
Triceps, 158, 169
Triceps Stretch, 184, 185
Two-Arm Row, 197

U

Unsaturated fats, 74
Upper Back Stretch, 185
Upper body strength, 148, 151

CHANGING THE NORM

V

Vegetables, 97, 98, 107, 108

W

Walk-Ups, 232
Weighing, 30, 145, 147
Weight scale, 98, 144, 145

Made in the USA
San Bernardino, CA
22 June 2017